Making
CANNABIS
PERSONAL

Take the Guesswork Out of Your Cannabis &
CBD Experience by Tailoring it to Your DNA

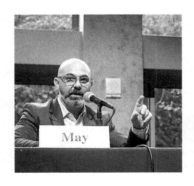
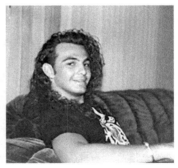

LEN MAY
with
O. BRIAN KAUFMAN

ISBN: 978-19-5-315341-8

Published by

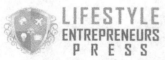
LIFESTYLE
ENTREPRENEURS
P R E S S

If you are interested in publishing through Lifestyle Entrepreneurs Press, write to: *Publishing@LifestyleEntrepreneursPress.com*

Publications or foreign rights acquisition of our catalog books.
Learn More: *www.LifestyleEntrepreneursPress.com*

Printed in the USA

Contents

CONTENTS

Acknowledgements

I have so many people to thank for where I am today. In case I missed somebody, I apologize in advance.

It's been an incredible journey so far, with many ups and downs, but I would not change a thing.

First, thanks to Brian for understanding my ramblings and helping me organize my thoughts into the book you are reading today. Next, my business partner, Eric, for supporting me through this process during Endocanna corporate time. My partners in Litt and Kush Kingdom, I thank for the things I learned working with you. Thank you to the people who mentored me at Medicinal Genomics.

Thank you to the team at Lifestyle Entrepreneurs Press and to Founder and Publisher Jesse Krieger for taking on our special project. Senior Editor Zora Knauf deserves much thanks for guiding us through the editorial process.

I am lucky to have many friends, and I appreciate the support of my Los Angeles crew: Anya, Kimberly, Mike, and Jerry (who brought Skye into Sasha's life). My Philly friends, who I grew up with, got me here, so thanks to Eric, Steve, Jim, Mark, Alex, Jen Azaria, and the rest of the knuckleheads. Closest friends—Mitch, Alex, and Steve— I appreciate all of you for always being there unconditionally. And to my new friends I met and built bonds with over at Dr. Michael's house, I look forward to more adventures with all of you.

ACKNOWLEDGEMENTS

Thanks to all the people whose paths crossed mine, people who worked with me to understand this amazing therapeutic plant called cannabis. All have inspired me, and I hope my accounts have done justice to your stories of hope and strength. All my mentors who I haven't met but greatly inspired me like Howard Stern, Raphael Michoulam, Richard Branson, and Elon Musk, I thank for showing me the way. And thanks to the Dalai Lama, who I really felt a connection with at his birthday party not long ago. Thanks to Lana, my ex-wife, who asked me to move to California where I found the opportunities in Los Angeles that put me on the road I'm traveling on.

My parents, who not only brought me into the world but also to America to pursue a better life, I thank you and all the rest of my family: Alex, Sofia, Alina, and Brandon.

Most of all, I want to thank my daughter, Sasha, because her light illuminated the meaning and purpose in mine. In addition to helping other people, she was able to help me break down my walls, which allows me to lead with love today.

When you connect in a loving way, it creates compassionate empathy, and that energy is attractive to everybody around you. When you put that out in the universe, it actually elevates everybody else as well. The hardships, abuse, financial insecurity, emotional toil, and everything else that has happened to me all were used as motivation to connect to an overall sense of purpose—my big why. It helped me make an impactful difference in people's lives. I hope everyone on their paths to healing can find that purpose too.

For Sasha and Jacob

Make
CANNABIS PERSONAL
FOR YOU

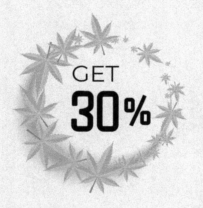

GET
30%

OFF YOUR DNA TEST
+
YOUR FIRST PERSONALIZED
CANNABIS PRODUCT
FREE

Preface

My interest in cannabis began when I was a teenager, and it never ended. I was so passionate about it that people even turned away from me; all had their reasons. Many of them thought cannabis use was wrong, basing their beliefs on moral or political ideas. Even today there are people who do not accept that cannabis has medicinal uses. Such thinking underestimates the true benefits of this ancient medicine. *Making Cannabis Personal* is meant to educate people on how cannabis is helping the human species find wellness and remove the ridiculous stigma and beliefs associated with it, such as "but people who use cannabis are just criminals or addicts." People use cannabis therapeutically and benefit from the medicinal properties of cannabis in unexpected ways. That's what this book is about.

You will discover amazing stories from some of the many clients I have helped. Each person from these stories who uses cannabis for wellness has a different experience. And it all starts with their genetics. Your DNA is personal to you. Cannabis responses are based on each person's genetics, so the responses are personal too.

I devote several chapters to explain how genetics interacts with cannabinoids to create truly unique experiences. I chronicle how many different people found treatments to recover from illnesses and alleviate conditions that afflict them. You may notice similarities between your experiences and the stories of my clients, like Jim, a vet suffering PTSD who found pain relief that helped him get off opioids.

Or like Grandma Mary, a woman suffering from side effects of chemo who found relief without feeling side effects from cannabis use. Both found comfort in specific CBD formulations that were tailored specifically to match their individual DNA profiles.

Writing this book is also a way for me to inspire readers by telling the stories of how everyday people found solutions. My own story is included: how I went from being broke and homeless to being a popular presenter at international conferences. This book chronicles how I turned my passion into a career. I talk about my early entrepreneurial days on the street, the laboratory hours spent testing and classifying cannabis strains, opening and running dispensaries in SoCal, and then building a biotechnology company committed to helping consumers find cannabinoid products that enhance their health and wellness.

As CEO of EndoCanna Health, I help others discover how to use cannabis to better their lives. Cannabis is therapeutic. It affects everyone differently; that's why cannabis is personal. But before I get to any of that, let me recount a story that opened my eyes to the promise of cannabis and its obvious benefits—an idea I have believed in since I first started getting high. Or, as was often said when I was younger: "Check this out—it will blow your mind."

First Thoughts

"The wound is the place where the Light enters you."
—Rumi

"Do not go where the path may lead, go instead
where there is no path and leave a trail."
—Ralph Waldo Emerson

"The meaning of life is to give life meaning."
—Viktor E. Frankl

Meeting Elvy

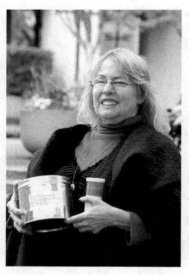

Many people know of Elvy Musikka. Born in 1939, Elvy became a national champion of medical cannabis use after being acquitted in a case in Florida, where she was on trial for illegally growing marijuana. In that case, Elvy never denied growing or using cannabis. In fact, you could see it in her glazed and bloodshot eyes! She used cannabis in an effort to counteract glaucoma, a progressive disease which left her nearly blind.

Elvy turned in desperation to growing pot after a 1971 study titled "Marihuana Smoking and Intraocular Pressure" reported that subjects who smoked cannabis reduced their glaucoma symptoms by nearly 30 percent. The study suggested that cannabis could work to relieve glaucoma symptoms when conventional medicine failed to help patients and when there were no other options.

In 1976, Elvy's doctors suggested she begin smoking pot to slow the progression of the disease. The doctors at that time, of course, could not authorize or prescribe pot use; it was a federally outlawed drug (and still is as of this writing). So, Elvy took matters into her own hands and began to grow weed in her backyard so she would not have to buy cannabis from black market drug dealers. It was a risk, but it was that or go blind.

Elvy was arrested after a neighbor complained to police, and she faced the possibility that she could be sentenced to five years in jail for growing plants that could save her life. Her attorney argued that Elvy's pot use was a "medical necessity," and her subsequent acquittal in 1988 paved the way for the medical community to begin to use cannabis to treat glaucoma patients. After her acquittal, as reported in the *South Florida Sun Sentinel*, Elvy said the thought of going blind was "more frightening than going to jail." So, she took the risk to grow medicine that was not legally authorized but was known to work. She said then that she did not believe "the law has the right to demand blindness from a citizen."

Elvy was not a stereotypical resistance fighter. She was simply born with congenital cataracts on her eyes and eventually developed glaucoma from that condition. Glaucoma is the leading cause of blindness in the United States. Elvy had some 14 eye operations since childhood and today still has little sight in her right eye as a result of surgery.

There's more to Elvy's story, and our stories are connected. She was one of four surviving patients enrolled in the Compassionate Investigational New Drug Program in the late 80s, which allowed her to get marijuana from the federal government. That program is infamous. The legal cannabis cigarettes that were available were of poor quality—machine-rolled leaves, stems, and seeds—and came from a federally controlled farm at the University of Mississippi, which has been growing cannabis for experimental purposes since 1968.

Since Elvy became one of the first four recipients to receive federally approved cannabis, produced by the feds, her story became famous. Then, using her notoriety, she became involved in the cause to support the use of medicinal cannabis for others. In fact, for her efforts, Elvy Musikka was named *High Times* magazine's 1992 Freedom Fighter of the Year. Today she resides in Eugene, Oregon and serves on the board of advisors of Voter Power.

I came to know Elvy from my role as President of the Cannabis Action Network, an organization that has worked to decriminalize and normalize cannabis use for both medicinal and recreational purposes. Today Elvy and I continue to stay in touch as we both work to decriminalize cannabis use and to legitimize the medicinal benefits of CBD and THC.

Taking Action for Cannabis

My story and ongoing journey into the field that promotes the use of CBD, and THC is a long one, and it begins long before marijuana use was decriminalized in many parts of the United States.

I met Elvy fighting the good fight to reconstitute the efficacy of cannabis. Since I was young, I was an advocate of medicinal cannabis, believing that nature provided a substance that was beneficial to people in many ways. This advocacy led me to a group which promoted cannabis use. It was called the Cannabis Action Network, and after only a short time working with its members, I was asked to be its president. In this role, I met many of the thousands of people working to legitimize the cannabis industry. Elvy was one of those volunteers. Her story, her condition, and her fight to win the right to use cannabis medicinally always moved me. And there were many like her who literally became test subjects when marijuana as a medicine began to gain both efficacy and legitimacy.

As chief of the Action Net, I was responsible for organizing and running rallies and seminars to build support for legitimizing cannabis use. A labor of love, for sure, since cannabis helped me focus and channel my own creativity. In my role as the chief lobbyist and organizer of CAN, I arranged for a large rally at Independence Hall in Philadelphia to attract support for our cause. What better place to fight for freedom than the place where our Founding Fathers gathered to write the U.S. Constitution? I invited Elvy to be our keynote speaker.

Elvy stood there—on federal property, in front of federal law enforcement, in front of the park's rangers—and freely, without concern for retribution, lit up a joint and smoked it. I thought, *This is how it should be.* This was my first epiphany. I knew then, believed then, that someday people in this country would come to see marijuana as medicine that could save lives.

Watching Elvy take care of herself looked normal, but—looking around, seeing federal rangers at the site—it did not seem like a good idea. Elvy could consume cannabis on federal property—right in front of federal rangers. If I did that, I'd be in jail. It was a visceral moment. Unreal.

There is another moment I will recount from that rally in Philadelphia. My most powerful aha moment—the moment where I saw with my own eyes why cannabis legitimization was needed. The night of the rally in Philadelphia, Elvy was a guest at my house. That morning, after a night's rest, Elvy was moving about in my living room when she accidentally knocked over a small statue, a keepsake that had no real monetary value. Elvy was truly blind. She could not see, did not see, that statue, which was in plain sight. I was shocked because the day before she had some sight. But more so, I was stunned when not long after she knocked over that stature, she had a few drags on a weak, federally manufactured reefer joint, and her eyesight returned to her.

In a few minutes, the veil of darkness that she had succumbed to in her sleep was lifted, and she could again see. With my own eyes I saw how medicating with cannabis instantly relieved the pressure Elvy experienced as a result of glaucoma. I had proof; I saw firsthand that what the Action Net and others were fighting for was right, was true, and that we would have to prevail so others could benefit as well.

As the army supporting cannabis use has marched on, the victories in the war for decriminalization began to favor those on the side of gaining legalization and fostering legitimization. Throughout, my involvement in the industry has taken many turns, and all of it has been rewarding. My background is intertwined with the story of cannabis legalization. Partly, that's because I liked weed, long before I knew that it could change lives and help people who were suffering from medical conditions and ailments. Today my appreciation and conviction for what cannabis can do is stronger than ever. As CEO of EndoCanna Health, I use the knowledge of the plant to help modulate the experiences of those looking to incorporate cannabis into their lives.

My Early Years

America is a land of immigrants, and I'm just one more. My co-author, Professor Kaufman, on the other hand, describes me with a word: "Original." I think that is high praise from a guy who doesn't get high.

Here's my story. I was born in Lithuania to a Jewish family at a time when Jews were living uncomfortable lives in the Soviet Union and its satellite countries. I was an only child of two tough people who were struggling to get out of our native country. My father was a hard man who sometimes turned to a belt on me to keep me in line. Apparently, I got out of line a lot.

We left the Soviet bloc country when I was six, making our way to Poland, then Austria, and finally we settled in Italy for a while, where my parents found work. Jewish refuseniks were being granted asylum in many countries, but my parents were looking for permission to come to the US, and when it came a year or two later, we landed in Philadelphia.

In Philly, we lived in a basement apartment on Foster Street with my grandparents, an uncle, and his family. It was a poor, tough neighborhood. On the streets, kids were looking to beat up other kids. At home my cousin beat up on me. I was living the American Dream.

As immigrants, we struggled to put together lives and livings. We had no money. My father would take me out, and we would drive around, looking to pick up furniture that was tossed out onto the street. He would repair and sell old TVs and anything else discarded. My father would always rant that "Americans throw out good things."

In Russia, Jews were persecuted and not allowed to grow our families and communities (which is why my parents only had one child). In the US, I was no longer seen as a Jew; I was looked at as a Russian—the enemy. This was during this time when the US boycotted the 1980 Olympics because the Russians had invaded Afghanistan. Being Russian meant I suffered through a lot of teasing, which led to a lot of fights. That history followed me: turmoil and fights.

We eventually moved to a house, and I started to make friends—people I'm close with to this day. Only children are loyal friends. Meanwhile, at home I still had a turbulent relationship with my father. My grandfather was ill, so my mother was busy taking care of him. I was left to my own devices—literally. The device was a transistor radio. On it I could listen to rock and roll, and music became an escape.

When I could not sleep, I would listen to the radio. I would record music from the radio onto a portable cassette recorder and make mixtapes. I would literally record a song off the radio onto a cassette, then would cut the tape and Scotch-tape it back together. Kids, right? But my mixes were good; people liked them. My mixes flowed. I was learning to be a DJ, although at the time I didn't know it.

My early favorites were, of course, the legends of rock: Beatles, Led Zeppelin, ACDC, Aerosmith, and the darker metal of Black Sabbath, Judas Priest, and Iron Maiden. Then I found hip hop. I watched the film *Beat Street*, and my life changed. It was one of three turning points (the time with Elvy was another, and another was the realization that genetics and cannabis were interconnected).

From that moment on, I was living on Beat Street. That became my life movie. My friends and I would try to act that out. I started imitating that lifestyle, wearing sweat suits instead of jeans, high tops instead of Vans. Everyone knows that look. That was my look. I still like that look. Ah, but *I was so much older then, I'm younger than that now.* (Sorry. I couldn't resist. After all, I'm talking about music too, and Professor Kaufman is a big fan of that Nobel Poet Dylan.)

Music has always been a thread. It was medicine. It was the one thing that allowed me to hold it all together. It was the one thing that made sense, and it allowed me to escape my family, the mean streets of Philadelphia, and my own crazy thoughts. When I discovered cannabis, it really blew my mind. Not to get too far ahead, but it was that *missing* piece—that puzzle piece that reveals the entire picture.

Here's how it happened. In eighth grade I was smoking cigarettes—you know, trying to be all cool and everything. Then someone gave me a joint. The immediate effect was that it slowed down my brain. I had ADD. This stopped that condition for a short while. With ADD, it's like your brain is a computer browser with a couple dozen different tabs open. Cannabis closed the tabs, allowing me to focus on the one tab that was open.

There are many ADD medications. Some make you anxious; others make you stupid. None are very helpful. But I found I could replace meds with cannabis. I have been on a mission to find the perfect cannabis profile ever since.

After that first cannabis experience, it became a regular thing. It was medication and it worked. I remember my friends would come over, and we would get high, watch *The Song Remains the Same*, and hang out until my parents came home.

Later, a driver's license meant freedom. I was out all the time. That did not help me in my relationship with my dad. We had some major blowouts, both verbal and physical.

With wheels and some nickel bags, I made my way around Philly. A fake ID then opened up a new world of clubbing. I was exposed to more music. And there was alcohol, psychedelics, cocaine, and ecstasy. I was careful. I knew a person could easily get hooked. For me, that stuff was recreational. Cannabis, on the other hand, was medicine.

I was always hustling, always going out. When I came home at three or four in the morning, I would grab a pole and then go fishing until noon. Then I would sleep all day and go out clubbing again at night.

Eventually, my parents went through my car, found my weed, called the cops on me, and kicked me out of the house. I was hurt but understood that my parents were too old to be part of the counterculture that took root in the late 1960s. I spent the next few months couch surfin'.

I eventually got my own place. My grandmother gave me money to get a room. It wasn't much. I could only afford a basement apartment. Every time it rained, my apartment flooded. I had a Shop Vac to vacuum up the roaches. There were six people living in the apartment above me, and they had dogs who defecated in the hallways. It was a nightmare. At that time, I kept thinking that I didn't want to end up destitute, looking for change in my car to get gas or buy gas station food.

Everybody has a choice. There's a way to hustle. With the right determination and desire—when you make it a must—you burn the boats. There's no way back. Motivation for not living in shit keeps people hungry and humble. And I made a decision to get out.

I sold weed. I got a job at Tower Records. I became a DJ at a strip club—called The Catwalk. Three jobs basically. But I was able to make it work. I even attended college and began working towards a degree in physical therapy. (Even then, I wanted to help people get well.) That work provided me with a good background in anatomy and physiology.

From being in that hell hole, the literal basement of my experience, I learned that I had to make a life for myself. I was able to get a better place. I was able to go to school. And friends would come over to my place, and we would listen to music and escape into the weed. OK, I didn't finish earning that college degree. I had sixteen credits left when I realized I did not want to be a physical therapist. I had more interest in business. So, I left school for a steady job.

I was happiest when I worked at Tower Records. It was music, my first medicine of choice. My job was to sell records, of course, and I did that. I was also involved in hooking up customers to my cannabis connections. I made money at both. I was rolling—rock and rolling, actually—and did well making money at my hobby. And I was young.

When I went to Temple University, I had taken some business courses. Now I was an entrepreneur, on a small scale, of course. I was known for having good stuff. One friend said, "There is a difference between down the way weed and Len May weed." He and others knew what that meant; I had an eye for the good stuff. A good reputation went far.

I became more interested in cannabis the more I was involved in selling and distributing it to my friends. I wanted the best and thought my friends would too; that was my mission. Score well, right? In this way I started my own research. I read the magazine *High Times* and was always interested in its articles that broke down the types of cannabis and various types of plants. And I read *The Emperor Wears No Clothes*, a non-fiction book written by Jack Herrer. That book was instrumental for many legalization advocates like me. But equally important, Herrer talks about the medicinal uses of cannabis.

From this book, and when doing a research paper in college, investigating reasons for legalizing hemp and all its cousins, I learned about terpenoids, flavonoids, and cannabinoids; about the science surrounding these plants. I knew about indica and sativa, but the more I read and researched, the more I began to understand what I already knew: that cannabis was special

As consumers we all want the good stuff. I called it "Kind Bud." The kind you want. The stuff that's kind to you (these are my jokes). It's corny, but it was the 80s, so think of the clothes and the hair. These thoughts went hand in hand with that. I wanted the good stuff and would sell only the good stuff. I was in business so I could personally enjoy using cannabis recreationally. But that soon changed.

My Years in Corporate

After my years at school, I went on to successful careers in real estate and in venture capitalism at Price Waterhouse. I was adding lines on my resume and was becoming an expert in finance, business, and industry. Included in this work was learning how to develop online training techniques as well as offshore development. Like so many people during their early years, I was involved in so many different ventures.

More creatively, I dabbled in the arts, designing cigar humidors and my own clothing line. I even consulted by creating a business called Len May Coaching, where I worked with people to help them meet their career goals. I was a successful business leader and I had ADD. I called it Attention Deficit aDvantage. I helped others with it who, likewise, had to learn how to use the energy and creativity that comes with a brain that turns ideas out at a breakneck pace.

I left Price Waterhouse to sell commercial real estate for Keller Williams and later became a director for KW Communications. I was making quite a success in commercial real estate in Philadelphia, but really, like so many others looking West, I wanted to find a way to get involved in California and the fledgling cannabis markets there. The new gold rush beckoned me like the shiny metal inspired prospectors 150 years ago. I'll spare my readers a rendition of "Oh Susanna" and some banjo picking. There was an opportunity here, and I'm a believer in the idea that if you do good things good things happen to you. At the forefront of this thinking, was the idea that cannabis is a beneficial plant and should be seen as one.

Kush Kingdom

I went to California, still employed by KW Commercial Real Estate. California is not a reciprocal state when it comes to honoring real estate licenses from other states, so I could not work as an agent in my new home without first getting certified, which meant some time to take a few classes. Thus, I came to California as a real estate consultant. When doing this, I had a couple of clients who wanted to open an alternative healthcare clinic. Obviously, they wanted to offer their customers a wide range of products, including products made of cannabis. When they came to me, I saw that their paperwork was not compliant with state laws. I helped them get compliant, walking them through the paperwork, filing the right legal documents that allowed them to open their stores. My interest, personally, was to become part of the cannabis industry in California. The only realistic way for me to do that was to go into the dispensary side of things. To that end, I invested capital in this start-up operation, and my clients offered me a partnership.

That was how Kush Kingdom was formed. We were an early entrant into the dispensary side of things in California, and we quickly grew a model that allowed us to duplicate our early success and to open multiple dispensaries. Our partners included, among others, rappers and hip-hop artists. At Kush Kingdom, we created several brands of cannabis products. Our stuff was "off the chain." One was called Kurupt Kush, and the other was Method Man Blackout OG (named after famous rappers and my biz partners). That was back in

2008 and 2009. Back then I wanted to focus on medicinal cannabis and its beneficial properties. Of course, many of the people visiting dispensaries were not sick but were enjoying the new freedom due to California's relaxed regulation. In those early years, cannabis use really was largely recreational. Californians had their chill on.

Cannabis always opens doors. In the old days we called our cannabis adventures *trips*. We were all *tripping* when we were younger. But now these adventures are business ventures.

For example, way back in 2009 (OK, that was not so long ago), I was hanging out in Compton, California with Daz Dillinger, the hip-hop artist who was part of the Dogg Pound with Kurupt, Snoop, and other big names of the gangsta rap scene. Everyone was getting involved in medicinal and recreational cannabis, so our paths were crossing.

Daz lives in Compton, in this large compound. He has an amazing house. I was there and I was the only white guy at that moment. I was there because I had experience in business, I was an expert on cannabis, and I was a big fan of hip hop. So, we were doing business.

I have to laugh because one of my partners there called me "Suit" after a character in the television program *Entourage*. I was the suit in the room in comparison to the artists I was surrounded with. Don't get me wrong. These guys are the tops in their business. We would hang out, talking music and cannabis. They would pitch me business ideas because I was the suit and they wanted my feedback.

One guy I was hanging with was Kadillak Kaz. He played his demo CD for us and asked for feedback. He even wanted to know what I had to say. I was in *the room where it happened* (that's a line from the play *Hamilton*—couldn't resist). In the early dispensary business, everyone was learning what it meant to be compliant. Before then it was organized drug dealing. We all had patients. We gave out free products to people who really needed it. It was the beginning of the industry as we know it; although, back then, it was not totally official.

When I think back on moments like this, I think how fortunate I have been to go from being an impoverished immigrant to being a *suit*, a man respected for my ideas and opinions. When I think of those guys, I hear their music in my head. I'm bopping along to the beats from Industrial Records to the tunes of "What Would You Do?" "100 Wayz," and the hit "That Was Then This Is Now." That was *this*—this great moment and many others. It shaped what we have now, a chance to help others.

Working as a Cannabis Specialist

Kush Kingdom was short-lived. It started when medical marijuana was legalized in California but ended with police raids. This was a political bust—none of the workers or my partners were arrested). But the L.A. sheriffs closed us down. Entrepreneurs like me and my partners were going too fast for the regulators to keep up, and the state wanted to slow things down. Since our doors were shut, I had to look elsewhere for an income.

I turned my sights on developing products. I was in on one deal with Litt California. I'll spare the fine details but basically I met with an investment group which turned me down, but at that meeting met someone who wanted to invest in me. I then partnered with people at Litt California. We had to find retail space, and early in the cannabis industry in L.A. (it is still the case), it's hard to find commercial property for cannabis-related businesses (a banking issue). With Litt people we found a place where we could begin cultivation. We built a hydroponic indoor cultivation facility for cannabis. We also developed a delivery service using Uber drivers. Unfortunately, the landlord was difficult to work with, meaning the deal kept changing. We carried on, of course, believing we could be successful.

The plan was to grow good weed, for recreational and medicinal purposes. Our grower was a top-rated producer from the Midwest. He was expected to settle in L.A., but that didn't happen, and the first crop yield was lower than expected.

In addition, one of my partners had a really interesting adverse effect with cannabis. It made him angry and impulsive. There's a gene for that. This was the beginning of my understanding how cannabis use is personal. I talk about that in detail in the chapters ahead. That was a really interesting thing because for me, it is the complete opposite. It's a completely relaxing thing, as if I'm experiencing an infusion of serotonin. It's a boosting experience. Anyway, I only understood the adverse reaction a person could have long after working with that partner, but a seed was planted for me.

There were some other funky players too. But still we carried on. Before our second harvest, our plants became infested with mites and the entire crop was scrapped. That's where it ended. Our hydroponic farm was shuttered, and I went out again, looking for the next opportunity. In truth, the enterprise was problematic from the beginning. This time I was better educated, understanding more about growing and what it takes to produce good plants.

At the Cannabis Club

I made many connections during my time with Litt. MCO House was a private cannabis club. I was the education director and had a stake in it, along with the Litt people. My job, or task, rather, since I did this without pay, was to hold training sessions. I was glad to do it but needed to do more research on cannabis because I needed to build a full curriculum for the training.

In one training session I met a man named Danny, a body builder, and we would soon become friends. Danny became the trainer at MCO House, and on one occasion he brought in some filmmakers, from China. Through a director, we were introduced to Wesley Snipes. So I had a chance to hang out with the actor and the filmmakers and we talked shop about CBD, sativa strains, and other cannabis industry elements.

That night we were together, I had this vape, and it was a pretty intense mix, meaning that it was something like 60 percent THC. One of the guys asked if he could take some hits. He was on crutches and wanted some relief from the pain he was in. I passed the stick, and he started taking deep hits. I said, "Hey, man, you know, it's pretty intense. You may want to take it easy with that."

The filmmaker said he was good, said he was used to smoking.

"Okay," I said. "Well, I've warned you. Gave you a heads up."

Things got interesting after that, and an hour later, the producers from China actually bought the rights to make more *Blade* movies.

Maybe they would have anyway, but I thought that the connection was curious. The producers were going to make the franchise into a real martial arts vehicle, using the martial arts styles that are used in China. I'm not sure that the deal was helped along with the vape, but it was certainly part of the creative thinking that was going on. Maybe it helped secure the deal for Wesley.

Anyway, as the evening wore on, that producer on crutches was strung out and rather incoherent. I gave him some water and then gave him some CBD from a tincture. About 30 minutes later, he started feeling a little bit better. His colleagues took him home after that, but the story is a really interesting incident because it tells you that THC, even for an experienced consumer, has to be used mindfully.

THC can actually have a negative impact if ingested in a higher amount than what's needed for medicinal or recreational purposes. We all have a threshold of what our endocannabinoid system needs, where the deficiencies are, and what we know they are. We can actually activate our endocannabinoid systems with phytocannabinoids. If we do it with care, we can get the right amount that's needed for us to feel well and balanced.

When we take too much, then the body actually communicates and lets us know that it's being given too much. That's why I am such a proponent for personalization.

Now back to Danny. When he was training for Mr. Olympia, I worked out with him twice a day. The other guys who worked out with him were built like monsters, with muscles on top of muscles. It was ridiculous. When we would work out our legs, it was very difficult during the second workout because they were very, very sore. Danny asked me if, when I was doing research, I could come up with something that might help for that condition.

I knew my cannabinoid side really well, but I was trying to figure out what was going on with the guys during their second workouts. Pain is not too unusual a feeling for muscle after it's worked out because there's tearing taking place. In my research I considered aminos and glutamine, proteins that are the building blocks, and from there we came up with something that could work. Looking at the known science, we made a formulation called Recovery and gave it to Danny. It worked for him, and he started recommending it to his clients as well.

One day he asked me to meet one of his closest clients who wanted to find out what we were doing. It was Mickey Rourke. We all met up, and Mickey told all kinds of stories about his life, of a loft he had in New York, how he had crazy parties, and about his experience with cannabis. He told me that sometimes it makes him paranoid, so he wanted to know about the Recovery formulation because Danny was training him. Mickey wanted to know if Recovery would make him better. I told him to try it.

Some 15 minutes later, he said, "I'm feeling pretty good." Then he launches into a story about his face, his scars, and boxing in general. He's an avid boxer, a professional boxer, and he was in a bad motorcycle accident and had to have reconstructive surgery as a result. Then came a boxing match in Russia. He took some hits that opened up the scars that he had from the reconstructive surgery. He had more repairs in Russia that changed his entire face as you can see today.

Then he tells me that he signed up to box again. I think he was 63, something like that at the time, and the guy he would be fighting was 33—that's a 30-year difference.

"You know, you have to be careful—this guy's 30 years younger," I said.

Mickey said he had a strategy of how to beat this guy, which he began to show to everyone in the room. He showed his strategic moves on me. Jab, jab, jab. Then, with an open hand, with those big sausage fingers, he hit me in the side, like a basic kidney shot. That's right—I was knocked out with a body blow from Mickey Rourke. OK, it was a TKO, but it hurt bad. Luckily, I had some of that Recovery formulation. It helped. And I came away with a good story to tell.

At Work on Medicinal Genomics

I next found work in the cannabis medical field as a certified medical cannabis specialist at a company called Medicinal Genomics. In this job, I traveled around the United States and Canada, gathering samples of different plant materials, then taking them home to analyze in my lab. I was extracting DNA samples and sending them to Boston for sequencing. And from that information, Medicinal Genomics built the first library of cannabis strains, creating what became known as Kannapedia. I already knew so much about cannabis, but this work was really an advanced study course on the science of the endocannabinoid system. Sampling the various strains added to my expertise as well.

This came about after watching a video that featured Kevin McKernan—he was the first person to genetically sequence cannabis and founded Medicinal Genomics—and at that point knew that his work could help people determine how to best use cannabis products. It was a moment when I knew that I had support for my suspicions. Another aha moment when the loop closes.

McKernan was speaking at a conference in nearby San Francisco, so I called his office and asked if I could meet up with him at that event. I was told I could have 30 minutes with him so I flew there. That 30 minutes turned into a three-hour meeting. We each had information that could help solve some of the negative-use issues associated with cannabis. So, from there, I went to work with Medicinal Genomics. Kevin was its chief science officer and its founder, and he had formed the company with his brothers, Brendan and Brian.

I noted earlier that my job was to travel to different cannabis cultivators across the country. I had a mobile lab, and I would take samples of growth material and would extract DNA from plants, purify it, and send it to a sequencer in Boston. I was part of the team that started Kannapedia (see Kannapedia.net). MG created Kannapedia "to publish genetic information" and "to provide the identity, heritage, and chemistry of cannabis and hemp plants" they tested. Much of my scientific knowledge about cannabis was gained while working with the McKernans.

This expertise did not come easily. I spent many hours gathering cannabis samples for research and chronicling the various strains. This was empirical research. I was going full CSI on these things.

For a guy who is clinically diagnosed with Attention Deficit Disorder (ADD), one would think that this would be excruciatingly difficult. The person with ADD does not do well when it comes to gathering, collecting, classifying, recording, and delineating data. But the research meant the world to me. I was interested, focused, and learned to overcome my challenges to research and classify the strains of cannabis in the U.S. In a nutshell, the job was this: as a consultant, I would go around the country to extract THC and cannabinoids from the many strains of cannabis to gather data points and create content for Kannapedia.

I got a firsthand look at the many complexities and intricacies of the different profiles of cannabis plants, of the different levels of terpenes and cannabinoids. Weed smokers could always detect differences. Medicinal Genomics was categorizing the differences. The differences mattered.

This work mattered for so many reasons. One time, I was at a meeting with a group of doctors, discussing treating epilepsy in children, some with CBD and some with THC. The treatments were varied, and some of the kids improved while others saw their seizures return. This was another big aha moment—the moment when I became convinced that cannabis is personal.

I understood then that plant genetics made a difference in a person's response to cannabis and how a person would react to different amounts of THC and cannabinoids. I learned then that a person's genes played a significant role in relation to a plant's genetics. A person's genes could be modified by the genes of the cannabis plant. From then on, I became obsessed with understanding that role—the way genes affected the cannabis experience. And since then, I have continued to learn about the actions, interactions, and reactions of cannabis use. I have long been an advocate for the medicinal use of marijuana and have made it my job to understand the endocannabinoid system, the part of the body that doctors rarely consider when treating their patients with cannabis or pharmaceutical medications.

When I eventually left Medicinal Genomics to pursue other opportunities, I partnered with Dr. Alan Lawrence. He was a medical doctor who studied at UCLA, and he also has a master's degree in Human Nutrition and a Ph.D. in Psychology. I joined him in his practice and worked with his patients, many of whom were suffering from cancer, epilepsy, Parkinson's, MS, autism, and many other conditions and diseases. Together we created formulations that were tailored specifically for each patient. In this role, I applied my working knowledge while learning about how our formulations interacted with other medications and with the nutritional side of healthcare. I was learning what it meant to treat the whole patient. This work helped me to understand different cancers and autoimmune diseases and medication interactions—information I use today in my consulting practice.

Later on, I would be working again with Dr. Lawrence, helping him design a curriculum that would certify people working in cannabis dispensaries. This was pioneering work since many dispensaries were opening up in states where medical marijuana use was being legalized, and yet the people running those dispensaries had only basic knowledge of the plants and products they would be selling. I helped design the program that, in effect, licenses the practitioners who would be filling cannabis prescriptions. Our mission was clear—we had to provide a working knowledge to would-be practitioners who came from many walks of life, and we had to do this quickly. Hardest of all, we had to pass on knowledge that both Dr. Lawrence and I had amassed over many years. To do this, we built a curriculum and created online training courses. Our training was provided to dispensary personnel and medical practitioners who could earn continuing education units (CEUs) for completing the coursework.

These courses were designed to aid doctors in diagnosis and dosings, something few MDs had knowledge of when it came to understanding how cannabis works. In particular, the courses focused on 1) the endocannabinoid system in detail; 2) disease states in relation to the endocannabinoid system; 3) published studies that detailed diseases in relation to the endocannabinoid system. The point was to help medical practitioners understand the different traits of the endocannabinoid system and how cannabis affected that system. Today, my working relationship with Dr. Lawrence continues, as he serves as the chief advisor to Endocanna Health.

My work sequencing plant DNA, designing formulations and compounds in dispensaries, and educating myself on herbs and essential oils helped me design the curriculum for courses at Dr. Lawrence's Institute for the Advancement of Integrative Medicine (IAIM). When this was done, I took the courses. Becoming certified was a formality, of course, but more importantly, this allowed me to test and verify the designs of the courses to make sure they were comprehensive, rigorous, valid, and credible.

From this work, I have gained an even greater in-depth knowledge of genomics, cannabinoids, and terpenes and have developed a deep understanding of their interactions with the endocannabinoid system. On my walls at home I proudly display my certificates: a Masters of Medical Cannabis and an Endocannabinoid Formulation Specialist Certification, both from the Institute for the Advancement of Integrative Medicine course curriculum, which I helped construct. These areas of expertise include understanding the workings of the endocannabinoid system and how genetic expression plays a role in human experiences. Because of this knowledge, and in this specialized role, I am often called on by the media and public organizations to speak on these topics to help educate the general public about the healing powers of cannabis.

I had worked in dispensaries, and long after I had made a meager living selling pot to other young music and weed aficionados like myself, I was again dispensing products. Back then it was all trial and error. Medical cannabis formulations were mostly guesswork. That's one reason why Medicinal Genomics embarked on a mission to sequence the DNA of the various cultivars of cannabis. As any casual consumer knew, not all cannabis was the same. So, I spent much time working in a lab, trying to figure out how to customize formulations for individual clients. Early on we knew that people responded differently to the same formulations—and that meant something was at work beyond understanding the different strengths and types of plants being used. In the early days, before we developed our courses, dispensers like myself could not understand why two people with the same disease—a similar cancer, for instance—would have very different reactions and responses to our formulations. I realized there was a need to study the synergistic effects of how cannabinoids and terpenes worked together. Knowing this would help us figure out how to match different people to compounds that would work best for them. I realized I also had to study essential herbs and oils.

In my own way, I set out to understand the different parts of the plant. I wanted to know about the food, medicine, and supplements people consume, which obviously makes a difference in how they are affected by cannabis. I sought to understand nutrition better, to grasp how supplements like herbs and oils and vitamins were affected by genetics. I was also interested in how thinking—how a person's mindset—connects to well-being. Cannabis, food, medicine, supplements, vitamins, and physical activity were all pieces of information. Knowing the pieces meant I would have a better chance of putting the wellness puzzle together. In truth, I was using the clues to put together the puzzle of my own life.

This idea was illustrated to me personally when I went to see Dr. Shuang Chen, a herbologist who could make suggestions for non-Western treatments. Dr. Chen was an experienced medical doctor who had worked in China and Japan and was a registered herbalist in the US, as well as an academic member of the American Botanical Council and a member of the American Herbalists Guild. She is one of the few medical doctors who practices both Western and Oriental herb medicine in the US. Dr. Chen is best known for specializing in treating patients with fungal infections, skin disorders, and health issues using herb formulas. She's been practicing medicine for nearly 40 years and is the author of *The Guide to Nutrition and Diet for Dialysis Patients* (2013) and *Herbology in Three Traditional Medicines for Acne* (2011).

One day, a dozen years ago, I became ill—had a 103-degree fever—and I was getting sicker. Dr. Chen made some herbal remedy suggestions, which I took to heart. After three days using herbs and oils, I was essentially healed and was back on my feet. Since then, I have worked to become knowledgeable about the natural world and its bounty; in other words, the natural, organic substances that are available and work to heal people in alignment with their own natural immunities and disease-fighting defenses. We are just beginning to understand how wellness is personal.

All of these lines of work, the many jobs, and the high level of responsibility that came with most prepared me for taking a leadership position in the fledgling cannabis industry. Then came the big jump. Then came Endocanna Health. It was time to take my place as an industry leader.

A Company Called Endocanna

Starting a new company in the early days of the industry in California to some may seem like I was trying to cash in on the green rush, the new gold rush that reputedly had hit the state. But that idea is misunderstood. Being in cannabis was not the way to get rich quick. It would take time for the industry to develop. People in early years had the chance to help it grow, but that was not a guarantee that they would be able to develop successful business ventures.

After the dispensary business, I started diving deep into the science and understanding and learning as much as I possibly could about the endocannabinoid system. I was meeting with people a lot smarter than me. A lot of scientists. A lot of researchers found that the endocannabinoid system is much like salmon swimming upstream... The unique thing about this system is that it regulates all the other regulatory systems. So instead of getting information from a neurotransmitter, into the synapse, and out to the body, it does the opposite to get signals from our body upstream to the neurotransmitters. It makes modifications, understanding what's going on in our bodies to help to regulate different systems.

As my knowledge grew, so did the number of people coming to me for advice about cannabis. Patients, doctors, and activists alike all sought me out for my expertise and ability to suggest cultivars that effectively treated chronic health conditions and symptoms of illness or medical treatments like chemotherapy.

While spending time with medical companies and scientists who were exploring the genetic components of cannabis and developing a cannabis cultivar library, I saw a pattern. Elsewhere I had written about how I could collect ten samples of Blue Dream (a cannabis strain), and a few of them would kind of cluster genetically around Blue Dream, two more would tend to be on the fringe, and the rest were not at all genetically related to Blue Dream. Realizing there was more mystery to uncover, I started on a journey of trying to look at how human genetics and the genotypes actually affect the phenotypes and how they work together.

As a result of this work to understand the role of human gene expression and the endocannabinoid system, I co-founded Endocanna Health and set to work creating a DNA test that could identify cannabis strains most likely to help individuals. The result is a breakthrough DNA test powered by a patent-pending super-chip that analyzes unique genomic markers. The information from the DNA test is then turned into a report that gives consumers personalized information about their unique genetic expressions. From there it provides suggestions about cannabis formulations that match what's called individual Endo Compatibility—an intersection between your unique genetic code and the properties of cannabis plants. Each cultivar has a distinct ratio of CBD to THC along with a host of other cannabinoids and terpenes, each interacting with your body in a unique way (I outline this sciency stuff later). The personalized results from the Endo·dna tests are like nothing else on the market, offering consumers an incredible array of science-backed reports about their health and wellness.

Endo·dna promises more breakthroughs in understanding Endo Compatibility. When I give talks, I like to tell current and future customers that they can continue to expect groundbreaking new research and information about their unique DNA that helps them chart their own path to wellness. Endocanna Health is a biotechnology company committed to helping consumers find the right cannabinoid products to enhance their health and wellness. Using our breakthrough DNA test, Endo·dna, we empower you to take control of your health with access to a growing list of health reports that include suggestions for the best CBD and cannabis products that match your unique genetic code.

My work with this company has brought me some notoriety beyond what I was already building. In addition, it allowed me the chance to be directly part of the cannabis business in the way that I am. I truly pinch myself every single day going to work. Actually, I never think I'm going to work. I'm just doing what I always did. With where we're at in history, there is no other industry that has had the trajectory that the cannabis industry has in the last few years. We've gone from complete prohibition to it being legal in more than three-quarters of the country.

In view of that, my intention was never for my company to become number one. We wanted to build a company that would help people to avoid an adverse event with cannabis. You can have an optimal experience because cannabis is personal, and that's really, really what we want to get across to people. Everybody has a personal experience with cannabis, and two people can take the same exact thing and have a completely different result. Because cannabis is personal, everybody can have their own personal experience with cannabis and it can be a really good one.

Working with Tommy Chong

The title of this chapter makes my head spin. Tommy Chong. A classic comedian from the 1970s and 1980s who partnered with Cheech Marin to produce some of the most iconic comedy sketches from the counterculture. As a comedic duo, they are known for their "Dave" sketch (where the catchphrase "*Dave's not here*" comes from) and likely best known for the film *Up In Smoke*, a cult classic about cannabis.

I met Tommy when I was invited by a DNA testing company to work on a video with the legendary comedian. I visited him on the set where he films his talk show. I was not supposed to be a guest on the show but was asked to come by to help Tommy go over the results of his DNA report. During the show, Tommy called me onto the set, onto camera, and asked me questions about matching a person's DNA profile to specific products.

In this particular show, Tommy unwraps a DNA test, models the swabbing test procedure, and packages it up again to mail out. Then they cut to him looking over his DNA test results. He says the test shows "what CBD products are most advantageous for you to use."

He continues, "We're dealing with medicine to help any ailments or afflictions that you may have. It's important that you identify what problems that you have, and you can match them up with CBD solutions." He goes on to say, "You want to have the right medicine for the problem you have. The test is scientific."

Tommy notes in the video that his test results suggest he has a little problem with insomnia. "I have a CBD product to help me sleep, and they say I also have a little inflammation, which I do, because I play golf and dance a little tango." He mentions he has anxiety because he's married to a beautiful woman—the fact that she is so beautiful is what causes him so much stress. The man's still funny. He then talks about the testing procedure and the products he's taking for pain and inflammation and to relax.

"The test will help you find the solution to your problems," he says. "There's exact science now. You don't want to mess with CBD. If you guess wrong, you can suffer needlessly." Then, to my surprise, he calls me up to explain how CBD formulations can be matched to a person's genetic profile. I went over his results and gave him insights into his DNA and how it affected his cannabis use.

Growing up watching *Cheech and Chong*, I never would have imagined that I would meet one of them. And to work with them—that would have been crazy thinking back in the day. So, when I knew I was going to meet Tommy, I brought along their first, self-titled album, *Cheech and Chong*. I never ask for autographs. Not usually. But I had that first vinyl album. It was a collector's item even without his sig. He was very excited to sign it. He said he appreciated that I brought it along. Tommy still has millions of fans. He gets it, gets that he is an iconic celebrity from an earlier time when cannabis use was widespread but not legal.

The joke back then was that the criminalization of marijuana was a joke. A sad one. It was a political football, and it created crime because people took risks to get and use cannabis. But times have changed.

Cannabis gets me close to people that I always looked up to—role models or people I have been fans of in earlier times. My interaction with celebrities and business leaders is all for a good reason: I'm helping people get well and working with people to build this industry.

Tommy has a show promoting cannabis and the industry. The company he was promoting, New Coastal, sells Endocanna Health kits and our formulations. Tommy says he's a fan, which is funny because I was always his fan. Full circle, right? Maybe we can get an act going: *May and Chong*. OK, maybe not.

Tommy Chong definitely found the information from his DNA test was useful. Our tests validated the information he had. After the show, Tommy even invited me to his house to go over the test results in more detail. I'm not saying I partied with Tommy Chong. Not saying. But I was there.

My experience working in the *corporate world* with Tommy Chong is a result of the changing attitude in this country towards cannabis. Cannabis is no longer a recreational drug used by those embracing the counterculture. Because of Elvy and the many people working to normalize marijuana, things began to change. Then came Colorado. Other states followed. And one day—maybe by the time this book goes to press—federal laws in the US will finally change.

For people who are ill, and there are many, there is new hope and help. Cannabis has life-enhancing properties. Many symptoms associated with many diseases can be alleviated with the medicinal properties in CBD and THC, two of the main active ingredients found in cannabis.

Cannabis can be used for wellness. However, finding the right cannabis formations that work in effective and safe ways is not necessarily easy. Many people became frustrated because cannabis was offering help, but it was inconsistent. When people began using cannabis for wellness, they discovered that when they went to another dispensary to find the cannabis that helped them, and even when they bought the same product, it did not have the same effect. The results were sometimes good and sometimes were not. I hyper-focused on this problem. I wanted to find a way to resolve this. All along, I have been involved with cannabis, each year becoming more active in organizations and businesses related to what was becoming a bumper crop industry in Colorado and elsewhere. And that's when I saw a problem that could affect the industry as a whole.

Cannabis in Ancient Times

Medical use of both cannabis and hemp are deeply rooted in humankind's ancient origins. Cannabis was first used as a medicinal drug "in 2737 BC by the Chinese emperor Shen Nung, who "documented the drug's effectiveness in treating the pains of rheumatism and gout." In ancient Egypt, papyrus scrolls note that medicinal plants "were used to treat sore eyes and cataracts." Tomb raiders found "cannabis pollen...on the mummy of Rameses II," and cannabis pollen has been linked to "all known royal mummies" (Bryan Hill, Ancient Origins, 19 May 2015).

In India, cannabis has been used in Ayurvedic and Indian medicine for nearly three thousand years to treat many health conditions, including nausea and other digestive conditions. Many religious groups, including Buddhists, Naths, Shaivites, and Goddess Worshippers, have used cannabis in their meditation practices as a means to stop the mind and enter into a state of profound stillness, also called samadhi. Cannabis is mentioned in an Indian creation myth, where it is named as one of the five nectars of the gods and designated a "reliever of suffering." In the original myth, the gods churn the Ocean of Milk in search of Amrita, the elixir of eternal life. One of the resulting nectars was cannabis. In the Vedas, cannabis is referred to as a "source of happiness."

Hemp has a long history in China. At one point, it was so prized that the Chinese called their country "the land of mulberry and hemp.

Cannabis was a symbol of power over evil. It was found in emperor Shen Nung's pharmacopoeia and was called the "liberator of sin." Shen Nung is credited with developing the sciences of medicine from the curative power of plants. The Chinese believed that the legendary Shen Nung first taught the cultivation of hemp in the 28th century B.C. So highly regarded was Shen Nung that he was deified, and today he is regarded as the Father of Chinese medicine.

Hemp was used in ancient Japan in ceremonial rights and for purification with an emphasis on driving away evil spirits. In Japan, Shinto priests used a gohei, a short stick with undyed hemp fibers, to create sacred space and purity. According to Shinto beliefs, evil and purity cannot exist alongside one another, and so by waving the gohei, the evil spirit inside a person or place would be driven away. Clothes made of hemp were worn during formal and religious ceremonies because of hemp's traditional association with purity.

Cannabis consumed in ancient times was likely lower in psychoactive THC with higher ratios of CBD and other beneficial cannabinoids. Now cannabis is a consumer product, genetically bred to produce heavy THC content and maximum potency. Stronger cannabis is preferred by some recreational users; however, when used mindfully, it's very effective for medicinal purposes—for people with pain and inflammation and to relieve side effects of cancer treatments.

The Endocannabinoid System, DNA, and Cannabis

The endocannabinoid system is the primary regulatory system within our bodies. It regulates many different functions, including psychological functions, physical functions, immune functions, and digestive functions. In this system, we have receptors built into our brains and our bodies. The receptors are protein molecules in our cells. The molecules take chemical signals from outside and transmit that information from receptor to receptor until it reaches our brains, which control our endocrine and central nervous systems.

This is the science: cannabinoids—CBD oils and THC—affect the endocrine and nervous systems, but more importantly, they affect the functions of these systems in regulating immune responses. Understanding this will help you have a conversation with a medical practitioner, so you can advocate for yourself and find treatment options that are available beyond invasive procedures and manufactured pharmaceuticals.

I am not a physician, but I have spent many years in the cannabis industry as a researcher, and thus will pass along what I know. Some readers may choose to skip the more technical parts, so in this chapter, I'll offer a summary, and then, in the two chapters that follow, I'll get more technical for the wonks who are passionate about the scientific stuff. In addition, the illustration provided on the next page demonstrates graphically the chemical processes.

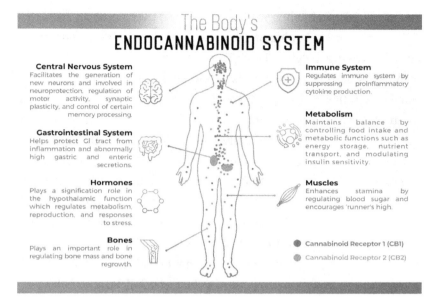

The Body's
ENDOCANNABINOID SYSTEM

Central Nervous System
Facilitates the generation of new neurons and involved in neuroprotection, regulation of motor activity, synaptic plasticity, and control of certain memory processing.

Gastrointestinal System
Helps protect GI tract from inflammation and abnormally high gastric and enteric secretions.

Hormones
Plays a signification role in the hypothalamic function which regulates metabolism, reproduction, and responses to stress.

Bones
Plays an important role in regulating bone mass and bone regrowth.

Immune System
Regulates immune system by suppressing proinflammatory cytokine production.

Metabolism
Maintains balance by controlling food intake and metabolic functions such as energy storage, nutrient transport, and modulating insulin sensitivity.

Muscles
Enhances stamina by regulating blood sugar and encourages 'runner's high.

● Cannabinoid Receptor 1 (CB1)
● Cannabinoid Receptor 2 (CB2)

This is the way the body works. Let's say that you stub your toe. Nerves send a signal of pain and discomfort to your brain. Your brain then sends out an immune response. The immune response is information sent out in the form of a hormone. These healing chemicals are sent out to address the information that something is wrong over in the stubbed toe. When you have your own naturally produced endogenous endocannabinoids, your body addresses that information properly with the right amount of healing chemicals, and then that pain and discomfort subsides and the information going to your brain subsides as well. When you don't have enough of your own endogenous endocannabinoids, you can get more of them from the cannabis plant.

The phytocannabinoids from the cannabis plant mimic the way our own endogenous endocannabinoids work. We have receptor sites that are already built into our bodies—CB-1 and CB-2—and these receptors take in healing information. THC binds directly with the CB-1 receptor site. A lot of the time THC can act as an analgesic (it's like taking a Tylenol). CBD, on the other hand, works as an immune-system regulator. This is how they work together. CBD reduces the inflammation; that's your immune response. THC works as an analgesic to reduce the pain. So when you're missing your own endocannabinoids, CBD actually goes and addresses those gaps in your own endogenous endocannabinoids to give you enough of the phytocannabinoids that actually replicate the way those endogenous endocannabinoids work. OK, that last part is getting very technical and wordy. The point is this: CBD recreates homeostasis—a steady state or chemical equilibrium. When you're missing endocannabinoids, you can get them from the cannabis plant, and that process creates the balance your body needs. That's how THC and CBD work together within your own body.

There's more. I will outline the process in more detail going forward. Most importantly, note this: everyone has a different genetic profile—a different set of genes. That means that no one has the exact same endocrine response to agonizing or antagonizing chemicals (to stimulant and depressant substances). So CBD and THC can affect different people in different ways. Some people are lactose intolerant. Some are gluten intolerant. Some are neither. People have differences in CBD and THC tolerances as well. Knowing how your genes are predisposed to certain effects when using cannabis will help you figure out how to make decisions in medicating in order to enjoy maximum benefits.

Our Endocannabinoid System — A Primer

Here's how it works. The brain controls the pituitary gland that secretes hormones to regulate the endocrine system. Hormones move through the bloodstream (a reason why endocrinal messages like hunger take several minutes to take space in your brain). The nervous system, on the other hand, is made up of cells, which are made of neurons. Messages that move along the nervous system reach the brain faster than messages sent through the endocrine system. For example, fear registers in the brain in a matter of seconds because it is sent as information through the nervous system. To continue, each cell's body (or soma) have dendrites—bushy branches which gather information—and these branches pass that information along to other cells. The neuron receives neurotransmitters in the dendrites.

On the other side is the axon, and around the neuron is a fatty layer called the myelin sheath. On the end of that are more spindly things called terminal buttons. When released, a hormone sets off an action potential—an electrical impulse that hops on the axon through terminal buttons. Terminal buttons then let off neurotransmitters that are next to the dendrites of the next neuron. When the neurotransmitters are released, they have to be the same size and shape of the dendrites of the next neuron. Space between the two neurons—synapses—pass along the information. Then the first neuron in the line performs a re-uptake—it takes back the neurotransmitter. The next neuron will only fire off an action potential if it gets enough neurotransmitters, and it fires off the action potential before the first neuron performs a re-uptake. These actions travel along the neurons to the brain.

Psychoactive medicines work on the neurons noted above. There are two types of psychoactive medicines: agonists and antagonists. Agonists bind to the receptor (dendrites), causing neurons to fire. Antagonists bind to a receptor but do not activate it, so they block the neuron from firing.

Along with those receptors, we also have ligands. Ligands are our own endogenous endocannabinoids that develop naturally and affect immune responses. And then, there are genes. Genes have a specific enzyme that affects how those ligands are expressed.

A Word on Terpenes

In addition to the above processes there are terpenes. The terpenes are the essential oils that the plant produces itself. The plant works synergistically with the cannabinoids and terpenes to provide a certain effect. Every plant has terpenes, essential oils, and these terpenes aren't just endogenous to cannabis. Regardless, terpenes are similar and yet different. Here's how to explain the way that it works. I'll give you an analogy using grapes, which are used to produce wine. Regardless of whether a grape is grown in Napa Valley, or in Italy, or in France, genetically, it's still a grape. But the way that you cure that grape, the barrels that you use, the humidity, the temperature, the heat, the light source, all that stuff, helps to express that grape in the wine, and the taste is expressed differently from region to region to region based on the curing method. That happens with cannabis. That's the expression of the terpenes. The way that you cure it will determine whether it's fully expressed and reaches its full potential. So the mix of cannabinoids and terpenes—and its expression—addresses the things you need in your body, and that helps to determine the effect that you're going to get. That is how a cannabis formulation aligns with your genetics.

So how does this work on the body? Here's an example about stress: We all have baseline endogenous endocannabinoids. My baseline level and your baseline level are different, so the way we deal with stress is different, and our genes have a lot to do with it. If both of us have different genetic profiles in the way that we experience stress levels, then something can trigger my stress levels differently than your stress levels. For some people, THC can produce a negative experience for cannabis users because their stress response will be triggered. When that happens, the brain will release cortisol, so their fight or flight response gets triggered. When cortisol is released into the bloodstream, it can create a feeling of anxiety or paranoia. That has a lot to do with our emotional response to stressors. And if I'm predisposed to that, then a high level of THC may trigger the fight or flight response. I don't need my fight or flight response in everyday situations; there's no jaguar that's chasing me that's going to pounce. All of a sudden, somebody cut me off in traffic, and I have this fight or flight response that I normally shouldn't have but I have it because I'm predisposed to that. That's an environmental trigger, but THC can actually trigger that in some people. THC can actually exacerbate that gene, and somebody can have a negative effect of that cortisol release due to a cannabinoid. But in addition, it has to do with a terpene profile as well.

Different terpenes, when combined with the cannabinoids, also have an effect on the body. So limonene, which is found in the sativa-dominant strain of cannabis, when combined with your cannabinoid, is supposed to give you a feeling of euphoria; it gives you a lift up. What it really does is boost serotonin and dopamine levels, but also it can trigger some additional cortisol into your blood. If you're already prone to anxiety and you're consuming larger amounts of THC, you can trigger that gene to express itself. And if that happens, and somebody needs cannabis for their medical condition, the results will not be positive.

Recently I consulted with someone who had PTSD, a veteran, and he told me that cannabis was not good for his PTSD. He said he can't consume cannabis because it gives him a feeling of anxiety every single time he uses it. He did not know what kind of cannabis he was consuming. Well, the first thing you should know is what you put into your body. The second thing to know is your genetic profile. It is possible to mitigate the expression of that anxiety-producing gene. So when we see that genetic profile and it shows that cannabis, that THC, can trigger that gene, and we also know the limonene can actually boost serotonin and cortisol, we know we need to mitigate that effect.

How do we do that? CBD can be an uptake inhibitor. It can reduce the efficacy of the THC. If you titrate up on CBD, it can reduce the efficacy of the THC, so it can limit the possible triggering of that anxiety-producing gene. For that terpene profile, instead of this "up" feeling that can create cortisol, what we want to do is create a more calming effect without a sedative.

In addition, we can look to linalool, which is also found in lavender. Linalool can actually support the THC to CBD ratio to produce a much more therapeutic effect that may not exacerbate and trigger that anxiety-producing gene.

The third thing is we can offer is another terpene suggestion. Beta-caryophyllene, which is also found in cloves and black pepper, is a really good anti-inflammatory. There is also an immune response when stress is triggered. And when your immune system is triggered, it usually creates inflammation of some sort. So, when you have a normal immune response—like when you stub your toe, which I talked about earlier—there's inflammation. But when you have an overactive immune system, the immune response is too great. You have unnecessary inflammation that you have to suppress. Beta-caryophyllene working with those cannabinoids provides an anti-inflammatory response. So together, that would be a formulation that is more optimal for someone who has a genetic expression that can trigger anxiety.

Then Comes the Metabolism

The important thing is to align your genetics with the right cannabinoid terpene profile. The second part of that is understanding your metabolic function—your metabolism. That is your method of consumption, how you dose, and what's appropriate for you. With cannabis, there's a certain amount of THC that can be really therapeutic, but if you take more than that amount, you can experience negative effects.

How do you know what's right for you? Well, your metabolism helps to determine that. There are ultra-fast metabolizers. These are the people who can have, say, a couple of drinks, and when the drinks are gone, they can take a breathalyzer test, and the alcohol won't show up. On the other hand, a different person can have a drink, they will be drunk right away, and a high level of alcohol will show up on the breathalyzer test. It's the same with food and everything else we consume. People can have ultra-fast, fast, average, or slow metabolisms.

When you are consuming cannabis, orally, through your digestive system, your liver, THC is converted to a different substance that is called Oxyhydroxide delta-9-Tetrahydrocannabinol, which is more powerful than THC alone. If a person's a slow metabolizer and they consume cannabis orally, it's a slower onset. There's also a much longer onset effect. Finally, the effect can also be a lot more powerful. A lot of people with slow metabolisms who consume edibles can have very negative experiences. They can have anxiety, paranoia, hallucinations, or even a psychotic episode. There are all sorts of side effects.

So, if we know that you're a slow metabolizer, we would suggest instead of consuming your cannabis through the digestive system, orally, that you consume it sublingually, under your tongue, or buccally, through your buccal cavity that's in your cheek, or through a vaporizer to bypass your digestive system. Then you don't have that chemical conversion occurring in the liver, and you can dose according to your metabolic rate, meaning that if you're an ultrafast metabolizer, you can take a little bit more. Not only can we guide you on what type of formulation is good for you; we can also guide you on what method of consumption is best and what dose is right for you.

Not only does your genetic profile affect dosing and formulation; the other things you put in your body have an impact too. Having a certain genetic predisposition doesn't mean that gene is going to trigger itself. It can be triggered by your nutrition, it can be triggered by your lifestyle, and it can be triggered by an event. So, all those things together give you a much clearer picture of how you're going to react to cannabis.

Your endocannabinoid system is the regulatory system, so the thing that you want to make sure you're doing all the time is maintaining homeostasis. And when something is off, the goal is to figure out what is off, what's creating that, and then work on recreating that homeostasis by using phytocannabinoids to fill those gaps.

On that same note, sometimes you have too much. There are people who have too much cannabis—too many endocannabinoids. So, they will have to listen to their body when it's telling them, "That's enough." In this case, you have to allow your receptors to reset themselves before you start consuming more cannabis—because maybe you don't need it.

Cannabis is Not an Opioid

If you want to consume cannabis recreationally, that's great, that's fine. However, in order to treat it as medicine, the goal is not to be on something forever. I previously discussed CB-1 receptors, where THC functions as an analgesic; that's the same receptor site where opioids bind to. That's your opioid pathway. So cannabinoids and opioids bind to the same receptor site. The difference is the opioid acts only as an analgesic. So when you have the signal of pain that I was describing before, it stops at that opioid receptor site, and you don't feel the pain. However, it hasn't done anything to address the inflammation that's causing the pain to begin with. So the opioid has no medicinal effect. But when you have the right ratio of cannabinoids and terpenes, it's addressing that inflammation. So you have the THC that's acting as an analgesic for pain, and you have your CBD and those receptors that are regulating the immune response to address that information and then recreate that homeostasis.

Your endocannabinoid system is a pathway that has a receptor sites in your central nervous system, your immune system, and your digestive system. There are other modalities that can address that pathway, but there's only one single plant in nature so far that actually has the phytocannabinoids and the terpenes that our bodies already have receptor sites built for, receptors that mimic the way those endogenous endocannabinoids work within our bodies. Cannabis is not a silver bullet, this is not a cure-all, but it is something that our bodies are already designed to use. The endocannabinoid system really is the system that allows us to maintain and regulate ourselves.

The use of medicinal cannabis stirs up plenty of controversy among healthcare practitioners and policy makers, as well as the general public. As more states and countries lift the prohibition on cannabis, many questions seem to be coming up like:

- Is it safe for patients?
- Has effectiveness been empirically proven?
- What conditions can it help?
- Are there addictive properties?
- How do we keep it out of the hands of abusers or high risk patients?
- What legalities should be considered?

I believe the answers to these questions start with your genes. Since the mapping of the human genome in 2003, thousands of scientific studies have been conducted to link genetic variants in your endocannabinoid system to a symptomatic condition. The challenge is to identify how those are expressed with the use of cannabis.

The clear conclusion is that a person needs the whole plant to work as a neuro-protectant. I started Endocanna Health to check genetic predispositions of cannabis users to determine what is right for each individual, including terpene profiles. There are numerous studies to support this, and an end to marijuana prohibition will foster new research as well as new and better strains of medicinal plants.

Thoughts on Cannabis Strains

I differ in my approach to classifying cannabis strains, as do others who are trying to create name-brand products in the industry. All cannabis is basically the same plant, but like people, the genetic differences are widespread. But people like to use the word strains. In truth, in the field of biology, strains refer to viruses. What we should talk about are cultivars and chemovars. The former is a cultivation variety, the latter a chemical variety. Ideally, we would be focused on the terpene profile and the genes of specific plants. Years back, we associated specific varieties of cannabis with the regions where they were grown. There was Durban, from Africa, and Maui Waui, and Thai and Afghanistan. Landrace varieties, and the differences were in cultivars and chemovars.

Say that ten growers are growing a variety named Salad Diesel. We can test their product to see if the genetic signatures are the same. Often there are marked differences because plants can intentionally or unintentionally change and mutations can occur. If a plant is cloned, it can forward genetic defects, and that, in effect, creates a genetically distinct plant. In fact, cloning a clone creates a higher chance of mutation—and many cannabis plants have been cloned.

So, in general, I do not embrace the idea of cannabis strains. Instead, I focus on cannabinoid levels and terpene percentages—on formulations—and the balance of CBD to THC in various products. Understanding that the ratios between CBD and THC is where the medicinal benefits lie and focusing on that drove me to find the differences in the products consumers use and the way those products are used.

My Father's Story

My father, who was skeptical about cannabis, is one of those people who found an effective use for its medicinal qualities. My father has arthritis. I told him I could help. I created a formulation that would bring down the inflammation from the arthritis and would alleviate the pain. When I think of this, my head explodes—but in a good way. This was the man I had so many fights with over the years. This was the man who called the cops on me, who kicked me out of the house, because of my involvement with cannabis. And here was a man who was now willing to consume cannabis. His thinking had changed.

The formulation my father was consuming had some THC in it. After a day of trying it, Dad said, "I don't think it's working."

I said, "Okay, so it's making you feel worse?"

He said, "No."

I said, "Well, if it's not making you feel worse, keep taking it."

He took it for another week, called me up, and said, "You know what? It's working. I really don't feel much more pain." That was an understatement. His hands were nearly nonfunctional before using cannabis. He couldn't make a fist. That was the before picture. After using the cannabis formulation, the difference was remarkable. Much of the function returned. His hands were stronger.

Then, when he went on vacation, he left the meds at home. But the pain never came back. And he became even more pain-free after that point.

My theory is this: the phytocannabinoids that he consumed stimulated enough of his endogenous endocannabinoids that they started functioning the way they're supposed to, and he reached that level of homeostasis where the inflammation went away. So, it's not, "Hey, let's take cannabis for the rest of our lives"; it's "Let's take enough so we can stimulate our own endogenous production. Then our bodies can start providing us with what we need."

The fact that my father was using a cannabis product is nothing short of a miracle. Before, my father had equated cannabis with heroin use. But later on, when he was sure that nothing else would help, he started to listen to what I said. I suggested he try Recovery, the formulation we developed for pain associated with workouts. It really helped ease his pain, and that is what shifted his perspective on cannabis.

In fact, my father's perspective on cannabis shifted so much that we ended up smoking a joint together while we were on a family vacation.

We do family trips every year. I take my daughter and join my parents. This particular year we met up in Jamaica. One day, my father and I were sitting on the beach, talking to a lifeguard there about ganga. The lifeguard's family had been growing cannabis for years. Later on, this guy brings me three different branches from his family's farm to try out. I rolled a joint and got high. And my father smoked it too. As the effects came on, my father did not know how to feel. I asked him how he was feeling, and he said to me, "Do you think we can get something to drink?" We did. And that was that.

A Medicinal "Life Saver"

Aside from help with the aches and pains of old age, as my father has experienced, cannabis can help people who are suffering from one of the most devastating of illnesses: cancer. Cannabis and cancer have been interconnected for a long time. Here's how the former helps the latter.

Sandy, a woman in her early fifties, was diagnosed with lymphoma. It is a cancer that begins in the lymph nodes and can affect the spleen, thymus, bone marrow, and other parts of the body. It is a bear of a condition. And not one that is easily dealt with.

Sandy was a wife and mother of two daughters. Her daughters were off to college, and Sandy and her husband were looking forward to this next stage of their lives—where they would have more time together to enjoy the comforts of middle age—when she was stricken with the disease.

Unfortunately, Sandy had to undergo treatments to fight the cancer, and as a result she was very ill from radiation and from chemotherapy. She was having a horrible time from the many side effects, including pain from her condition and the ill feelings caused by the drugs meant to make her better in the end. And, she was afraid—for herself, her husband, and her children. In fact, her eldest daughter was engaged, and Sandy was worried that she would not live to see her daughter get married later that year.

Like many cancer sufferers, Sandy had heard that medicinal marijuana could help her tolerate the harsh medicines that were fighting the cancer. Living in Texas, Sandy was prohibited by that state's archaic laws. Like Elvy and others before her, the medicines that could help save Sandy's life were off limits, legislated against because the organic treatments available were misunderstood or were being blocked for use by Big Pharma and other big money players. She was what I call a Cannabis Refugee.

"I was getting a strong chemo treatment, which almost killed me," she told me after Endocanna found a way for her to get help.

Before coming to me, Sandy's daughters managed to find her medicines to lessen the side effects of the chemo, but the cannabis she consumed compounded her feelings of anxiety, so much so that its use was not beneficial. She tried medicinal marijuana to alleviate some of the symptoms from the chemo, but the cannabis she was using made her anxiety unbearable. So, she could either feel pain or feel anxiety, and neither was a good choice.

When Sandy heard about Endocanna Health's DNA/cannabis testing, she ordered her kit and quickly learned from her results that she was genetically wired for a likely adverse reaction to cannabis. In other words, her genes suggested she would respond negatively to cannabis in the form of increased anxiety unless she used a specific THC/CBD formulation. She needed a formula that would align with her anxiety. After discussing the results of her genetic test, I suggested a specific formulation, which her daughters could purchase in California.

The formulation was a ratio that called for a very limited quantity of THC. Some was needed for her ECS system to reach homeostasis, but too much would trigger elevated feelings of anxiety. She did not want a high. And she did not want to feel anxiety. So, Sandy found a formulation that aligned with her genetics. The formulation was high in CBD and suppressed the THC levels of the cannabis. The terpenes that were selected for the formulation lessened the anxiety provoked by the THC.

This was more appropriate for her, as it would mean she would not experience being high and would not have increased anxiety from the THC. What she wanted most was to feel better and continue to live a full and productive life.

"It was a life saver," Sandy says. And that is not an exaggeration. In fact, it helped her in four ways: 1) She was super sick from the chemo, but the suggested THC/CBD formulation alleviated her nausea, tempered her pain, and even reduced swelling and inflammation; 2) it helped clear her mind, created a calming effect, and this different state of mind allowed her body to heal; 3) her consistent use proved beneficial, as it actually showed visible reductions in the disease on subsequent PET scans; and 4) she found a new purpose, becoming a supporter of medicinal cannabis and an activist for its legalization.

In Sandy's case, as it is with many others, any anxiety experienced easily could be the result of her cancer condition. I can only imagine the thoughts a person experiences, their concerns for family, and the fears inherent in suffering from discomfort, pain, and changing life circumstances. Such thoughts and feelings and fears can only make the suffering worse.

Sandy's is one of many stories of people who got help but who have had to go to great lengths to enjoy the benefits of cannabis because she lived in a state that does not allow cannabis use. To that end, she is now one of the thousands of people with similar stories who are part of the effort to lift prohibitions in Texas and a dozen or more states that still bar cancer sufferers from using an organic plant that has been shown to work.

Sandy not only lived to see her daughter married but continues to thrive today. Radiation and chemo were successful in treating her cancer because she could live with the side effects, which were dampened through the right formulation of CBD and THC.

A Returning Vet "Couldn't Cope"

Housewives, mothers with young children, and overstressed CEOs like yours truly are not the only ones who experience anxiety, and for many people, anxiety can be crippling. A three-hundred-pound NFL lineman has no worries when he is in the zone, immersed in a game. Same for the soldier in battle—he may be cool when bullets are flying because his training kicks in. But those kinds of high-pressure situations are not where anxiety attacks strike.

My friend Sebastian is a veteran who spent many years serving overseas in some fairly challenging environments. In those confused and chaotic situations, Sebastian is literally cool as a cucumber. But back home, on a pleasant sunny day, just the sound of birds chirping can elevate his anxiety to unbearable levels. "I couldn't cope. Sounds crazy, but the quiet makes me crazy," he says. Sebastian was trying to fix his feelings of unease by consuming large amounts of THC-heavy cannabis. And even without genetic markers for anxiety, that can lead to feeling overanxious and panicky.

I worked with him on his consumption formulations. First, for 30 days, he consumed only CBD-infused products. That allowed his receptors to reset themselves. Then we slowly introduced THC. We kept it low until Sebastian was able to safely raise the level to the point where he could realize THC's relaxing benefits. Today Sebastian knows to titrate down whenever he begins to feel anxious.

The important thing to do is to listen to your body. Homeostasis is about balance. When you feel balanced, you are at your best. Today, knowing this, and knowing that we can test a person's genetics to understand how susceptible they are to negative cannabis responses, means that we can help consumers realize the benefits of cannabis use, even when anxiety issues are a problem. Feeling anxious—like Sandy about an illness, or like Sebastian, who is settling into a quieter life, or for anyone suffering with an anxiety disorder—is no longer a barrier. Now these people can benefit from the right formulations of cannabis products.

My Roommate the Lightweight

In the old days, we were using cannabis recreationally to get high and to expand our minds. We would literally escape into our heads and the music we were listening to.

Back then, we would joke about lightweights—our friends who would get way too high and freak out after a few tokes or bong hits. Today, that's no joke, of course, but early on, we thought it was amusing. It was all part of the fun.

In those early years, I had a roommate named Mike, and we would hang out and smoke all the time. Every once in a while, if we smoked cannabis and then went out to see a film, or listen to music, or hit a club, Mike would have a panic attack. During these episodes, he would be sweating, would feel light-headed, and would have to sit down. One time he actually passed out. That was unusual, but it started to become a consistent pattern. It seemed to happen with a stressful event.

In fact, one of the first times I remember it happening was at a Valentine's Day party (when you're young, this is always a stressful day). The next time it happened, we were at a club, and I found Mike leaning on a column like he was drunk. He was drenched, both shirt and jacket soaked through. And again, at another club, we were hanging out, and he started passing out.

These social events were stressing him. I know now that he had a genetic predisposition to anxiety. As a result, he was scared to consume cannabis. If we were at home or watched TV, there was no issue. It was only when we were outside, doing something stressful—at least, that is my hypothesis. The combination of the stimulus and the kind of cannabis that we were consuming, without actual knowledge of what we were consuming, was the problem. We had no test results.

Growing up, there were times when people had adverse side effects using cannabis, so much so they stayed away from it altogether. I would have too. But that would also mean staying away from benefiting from its good properties, its medicinal benefits.

Mike did that. Gave up using cannabis. But then he tore his ACL. Painful. And an injury that requires surgery and a long recovery process. Mike told his doctor that he did not want to take meds but also did not want to be in extreme pain during his physical rehab. By that point, we know a lot more about cannabis and what medicinal benefits it offered. I suggested a tincture, a formulation for Mike, that would reduce inflammation and offer some analgesic comfort as well.

He was fearful, and understandably, given what had happened to him when we were young. He did not want to feel that adverse reaction ever again. Still, he knew that many people were benefiting from cannabis. I suggested a product, and he tried it and was fine and benefitted from the formulation. No adverse effects. None. Better than that, the medication helped Mike recover.

Mike's story is not unique. Many people have adverse effects on THC and swear off using cannabis as a result. But cannabis can be beneficial. We know more about it and how it affects people differently, and now we can match formulations to people's genetics. People who have had preconceived notions based on what happened in the past are realizing that those reactions are likely just a thing of the past.

A Survival Story

Today, we have a much better understanding of how cannabis can be used to alleviate painful sensations. It can work in two ways: it relieves inflammation, and it acts as a pain reliever.

I consulted recently with a woman named Deborah who had breast cancer and its associated pain. She told me she could easily go on about how hard it is to tolerate and about how much energy it consumes. She told me that pain exacts a heavy toll, and in most cases, it is paid for through the loss of joy.

Deborah was in her forties when she was diagnosed with breast cancer. About one in every eight U.S. women (roughly 12 percent) will develop invasive breast cancer over the course of their lifetimes. And for women, along with skin cancer, it is the most common cancer. Fortunately, the survival rate for breast cancer sufferers is high, but the treatment is not pleasant. For Deborah, this was the case.

Deborah experienced anxiety, nausea, and pain as a result of her chemo treatments, and then her condition worsened when she experienced the onset of adult shingles. Shingles is a painful viral condition that can affect the back, face, and other highly sensitive areas and is marked by a terrible itchy and painful rash. The condition hurts, but experiencing it while undergoing chemo makes it unbearable.

Pain is a signal sent to the brain through neurotransmission, which is the process of communication between the neurons in the brain. During neurotransmission, neurons and nerves send signals to each other through the use of neurotransmitters. These neurotransmitters release chemicals in the brain that tell us what to think and what to feel. The specific neurotransmitter that deals with pain is called a nociceptor. When we suffer an injury or any form of tissue damage, the neurons send signals to the brain, which releases chemicals in the brain to make us feel pain in the affected areas. These neurons will continue to release these signals until we introduce drugs to block the pain receptors, or until the tissue begins to repair itself.

Deborah, feeling pain from shingles, was suffering. Pain medication dulled it some but really had little chance of improving her day-to-day living experience. Deborah, of course, had heard that cannabis could help her feel better. But there was another problem: her husband was an alcoholic and drug user and had been living clean and sober for some twenty-eight years. Deborah was afraid to use a drug that could jeopardize her husband's sobriety.

When she finally came to see me about her pain and other symptoms experienced from her cancer and associated conditions, I understood her concerns. Many people have similar issues around cannabis use. They want the medicinal benefit but do not want the high that the plant is known for. To help ease Deborah's mind, as well as her pain, I went with her to a dispensary. I suggested she first try a topical cream—one that had CBD but only had a trace amount of THC.

The new medicine worked well from the very start. Her back pain from the shingles diminished from what she described as a level-10 pain down to a level 5. And later, she was able to actually sleep, which is something everyone agrees is hard to do when you're in pain. Pain pills did not really help with that symptom.

The next option for Deborah was a tincture—again, one that offered the benefits of CBD but only had a trace amount of THC. In my experience, a little THC, even a minute amount, is needed for someone to achieve homeostasis. The next day, Deborah called me because she was pain free. And from that day on, Deborah has been a true believer in the properties of cannabis. She survived the cancer and did so with less pain and less nausea. "I was hopeful it would work, and it worked better than I really expected. It helped me get past the pain," she says. As a result, Deborah became an activist for cannabis decriminalization. In fact, her husband joined the cause too. He is one of many individuals in sobriety who have come to see CBD use as something that can benefit those in pain.

Grandma Mary

Imagine a sweet old lady, your typical grandmother, doting on her grandkids. That's Grandma Mary. She could be anyone's grandmother.

If you have heard me talk at a conference, interviewed on TV or radio, or listened to my podcast on cannabis, then you have heard me talk about Grandma Mary, a woman who was suffering through chemo treatments for cancer and was having a tough time. The symptoms were bad, and the side effects worse. It's an all-too-familiar story in 21st Century America and elsewhere. However, one thing that would help her would be to use medicinal cannabis to alleviate the symptoms of her treatments. But for Grandma Mary, the choice to start that kind of therapy seemed out of the question.

Here's why: Grandma Mary was relatively hip back in her day, enjoying life and being adventurous. In fact, at a party more than fifty years ago, she tried a marijuana-laced brownie—something most baby boomers can lay claim to doing. She ate the brownie and, sadly, had a bad reaction, or as we used to say, a bad trip. Mary swore off cannabis from that point on.

But then came cancer and chemo and the unpleasantness that came with both. Nothing unique or different to what thousands of other fellow sufferers have undergone. For many, cannabis is something that can make treatment easier. To that point, watching CNN, Mary heard the respected Dr. Sanjay Gupta, a neurosurgeon and medical reporter, talking about the benefits of cannabis. And he apologized for his earlier position of discounting its effectiveness in treating people suffering from many diseases.

Dr. Gupta said, "I didn't look hard enough, until now. I didn't look far enough. I didn't review papers from smaller labs in other countries doing some remarkable research, and I was too dismissive of the loud chorus of legitimate patients whose symptoms improved on cannabis."

After hearing that, Grandma Mary, following a doctor's advice, decided to give cannabis a try. She went to a dispensary and purchased cannabis in chocolate edible form. She was told then by the dispensary budtender that she should start by trying only a small amount. So, she started by taking a small piece of chocolate, and waited, but nothing was happening. Then she started to feel anxious, she started to hallucinate, and the panic set in. Afterward, she again swore off cannabis and told all her friends at the assisted-living center where she was staying not to use it. "I thought it was BS," she told me. (Grandma Mary is a typical grandmotherly person, but she's also got a colorful side!)

The chemo continued, and Grandma Mary was stuck experiencing the awful side effects that came with it. I met Mary at this point and suggested she take a DNA test. She did, and the markers in her DNA suggested she was a poor metabolizer through her digestive system. This means even if she only ingested a little bit of cannabis, it would cause her an uncomfortable physical reaction. Brownies and chocolate were not the way to go.

The solution for Mary was relatively simple: she needed a cannabis formulation that came in a sublingual form. CBD/THC combinations taken under the tongue bypass the liver and, thus, are metabolized at a faster rate. For Mary this meant no unpleasant physical reaction. I helped her to her first positive experience.

Not long after, her appetite returned, and other side effects and symptoms were alleviated. Mary, like many of the people I helped, did not keep the news to herself. In fact, Mary became an activist, telling her friends and anyone else who would listen about her positive experiences with cannabis and how it helped her get through the illness she suffered from.

A Gallery of Pictures

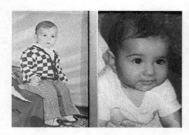

The author at age two; his daughter Sasha a year younger.

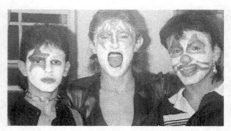

A Halloween Kiss cover band with friends featuring Len as Paul Stanley (left). Len created the band's make-up.

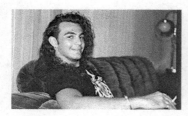

Len during his Tower Records days.

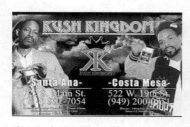

First Kush Kingdom ad featuring Kurupt Kush and Method Man Blackout OG products.

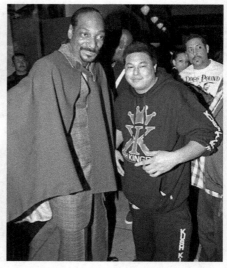

Snoop with Len's partner Mikey during the Kush Kingdom days.

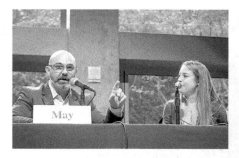

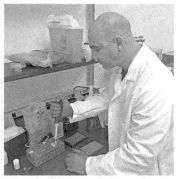

In the lab at Medicinal Genomics.

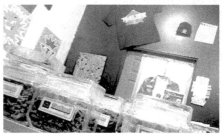

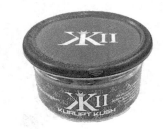

Speaking at the Digital Hollywood Summit in 2018 alongside the moderator Brooke Burgstahler (a news anchor for Marijuana Morning News).

Product at Kush Kingdom dispensary.

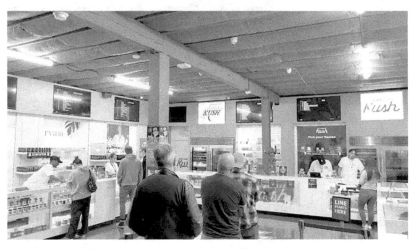

Business was good! A line forms at one of the Kush Kingdom dispensaries.

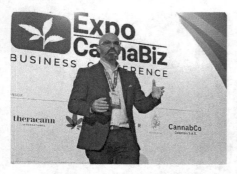

As CEO of Endocanna Health, the number of conference talk opportunities have grown. Picture at left is at Columbia's largest cannabis conference. Below is another "LENTalk" — this one at Cannatech in Cape Town, South Africa. (By the way, my co-author Brian Kaufman says he owns the LENTalk joke, but I think I have heard it before.)

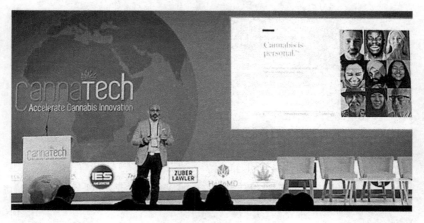

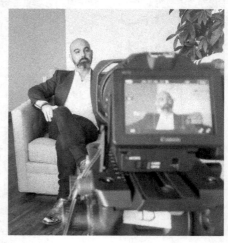

Taping an interview that aired on Japanese television. Cannabis is personal in places all over the world and in every language its healing properties are spoken of.

Hanging with Tommy Chong during a taping of *The Tommy Chong Podcast*. One day I'll have Tommy on my new podcast called *Everything is Personal*. It's available on Apple and wherever podcasts live.

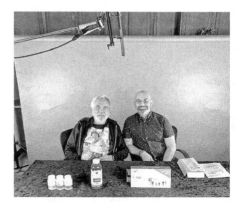

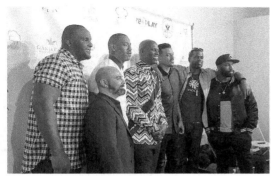

NBA basketball greats Glen "Big Baby" Davis, Kenyon Martin, Al Harrington, Matt Barnes, Stephen Jackson, and Baron Davis. I guess this is proof I'm not seven feet tall.

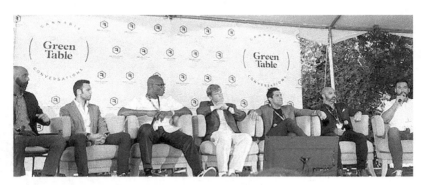

From the left: Jim McAlpine moderating a conference at Jim Belushi's house with ex-Philly Flyer Riley Cote, the NBA's Al Harrington, superagent Leigh Steinberg, UFC's Frank Shamrock, Len the "Sciency Guy" (that's what they call me), and NFL wide receiver Nate Jackson.

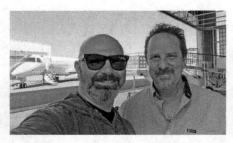

The brain trust. On the way to Vegas with Endocanna Health Vice President Eric Kaufman. We met at a cannabis conference and formed a partnership then and there to help people benefit from cannabis.

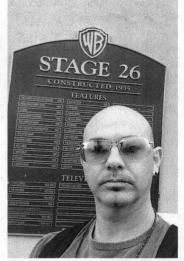

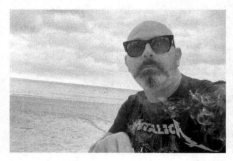

Chilling in Jamaica.

On the Warner Brothers lot working on the set of *Disjointed* as a prop advisor. It was cool to be on the set where the films *My Fair Lady* (1964), *The Great Race* (1965), *Gremlins* (1984), and TV shows *The Waltons* and *Two and A Half Men* were filmed.

NFL great Ron Brown hanging with me and Sasha. My daughter and I look a little different from those early baby pictures on the first page of this gallery. I don't have a baby pic of Ron Brown.

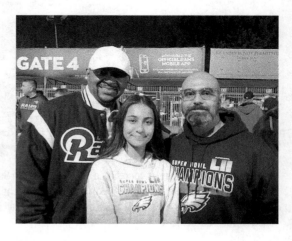

Hallucinations, Paranoia, and Anxiety

Some people have fast metabolisms. Some slow. As we get older, our metabolisms begin to slow down. One can eat only so many Snickers bars. This was true for a friend of mine named Allison. (I discuss how metabolism affects cannabis use earlier in the book – Allison's story is the perfect example of this effect.)

When Allison gets together with friends, she has to watch her intake if she enjoys cannabis recreationally, or on her own when she uses it medicinally. And she's a young adult, college age, so likely her metabolism will slow down even more.

"I cannot enjoy cannabis with my friends," Allison says. They have a good time. I get anxious. And it lasts forever. A little bit, and I'm in trouble." And when asked what happens, she says, "I experience hallucinations, paranoia, and terrible anxiety."

Allison's DNA test explains to me exactly why. Her profile shows that she has the FAAH gene, which breaks down anandamide—and that creates anxiety for anyone consuming THC. And she has the AKT1 gene, which means she is at risk for psychotic hallucinations when consuming THC. And lastly, her genotype profile shows she is a poor metabolizer of THC.

Cytochrome P450 and the CYP2C9 enzyme is responsible for metabolizing THC. Cytochrome P450 is a group of enzymes involved in drug metabolism and found in high levels in the liver. These enzymes change many drugs, including anticancer drugs, into less toxic forms that are easier for the body to excrete. The cytochrome P450 (CYP2C19) enzyme is one of the two main drugs with enzymes responsible for the metabolism of CBD.

Cytochrome P450 also creates the psychoactive 11OH-THC metabolite. After THC is ingested, your liver goes to work on it, converting it into other molecules in order to eliminate it from your body. These other molecules are called *metabolites*.

Allison has a genotype that is associated with being a poor metabolizer of THC. It means she may need a lower dose or maybe she can her first pass and consume sublingually. If she ingests THC that is metabolized through the liver, it can create an effect that comes on slowly, lasts a very long time, and is more intense.

That's a perfect storm. It means THC is likely not something that she should take, and if she does, it would have to be in minimal doses at best. Allison can still take CBD-heavy formulations. "My genetic profile says cannabis has to be used carefully, and I have to avoid edibles. I can still benefit from CBD. Glad I was tested. I now know what I can and cannot do." I was able to help Allison in the end. One way that Endo·dna was able to support her was by providing a suggestion for a formulation that has a slightly higher CBD ratio with a terpene profile that is Endo-Aligned for more linalool and less pinene (linalool has been shown to lower the adverse anxiety effects of THC). The other suggestion I had for her was based on metabolism; I suggested a sublingual delivery avoiding the first pass of digestive consumption.

The feedback was substantial. In a follow-up conversation Allison reported having a very positive experience and did not have an adverse event as she had previously.

People who consume THC feel the effects differently and in different magnitudes. It's not just a difference between the good stuff and second-rate cannabis. Part of the reason for this variability is due to differences in drug metabolism. The right formulation can correct any adverse effects resulting from a slow metabolism.

"You Can't Get Addicted to Pot"

How many times have we heard people say, "You can't get addicted to pot"? That's a bold statement. It's mostly true. But some people can become dependent on cannabis (specifically THC.) For example, people with the CNR1 gene can develop a greater dependence on THC.

The reasons for this are complicated. Of course, for those who face addiction, the complications are many. So let me break down how THC dependence works.

There are few stories I know relating to people who have had a dependence on drugs and alcohol and have used cannabis to alleviate their compulsion. People who come to me, and people I work with, generally are aware that cannabis contains chemicals that naturally work in concert with the body's endocannabinoid system. Unfortunately, as with anything, some individuals can go too far and may use too much cannabis with extremely strong concentrations of THC or use it to the point where they are dependent on it. It's a case of using too much of a good thing.

I know also that there are people who cannot make use of cannabis and its medicinal properties because it does not fit with their adopted sober lifestyles and maybe their moral philosophies. And, there are still others that have used cannabis as a virtual cure to stop drinking, as a way to relieve their alcoholism. In fact, I have been told that in the earliest days of Alcoholics Anonymous, many hardcore drinkers used cannabis to ease their cravings and temper symptoms of withdrawal from alcohol dependence.

One story that comes to mind involves a woman with a young family and a thriving career who was sidetracked by a medical condition. She turned to cannabis to relieve pain and other symptoms but got more than she had bargained for. I helped her negotiate a way out of dependence so she could enjoy the therapeutic properties of cannabis.

Being dependent on cannabis was one of the many concerns faced by Jessica, a woman in her forties who had children and a husband and who by all accounts should have been living a normal life. She had a professional career, but it was put on hold because she had a medical condition which forced her to go on disability. On top of that, Jessica was a long-time user of cannabis, having used the plant medicinally for much of her adult life to control the pain caused by her condition.

"I couldn't function anymore," she says. "I was disabled. I was stressed out. The panic attacks were horrendous."

Jessica was using cannabis to control the pain from her physical disability. Unfortunately, the medicine was making her ill as well. On top of it, she could not stop using cannabis. "Nothing made me feel good. But not using it made me feel worse. I didn't think I could stop. It felt like there was no way of winning."

After hearing me talk on a TV broadcast, Jessica came to me for help. "I was sure it was the THC that was causing my panic attacks," she says. "If I could stop them from happening, I thought I could get better. At least it would help me function better."

Working with her, we found a solution. I administered a swab test, sent out the DNA samples, and the report came back and showed us that Jessica was likely intolerant to THC and also would likely be dependent on THC. That's a genetic pairing that we sometimes see, and it explains why people like Jessica struggle using THC and also struggle stopping their THC use. So I helped Jessica titrate down over a few weeks, until we settled on a formulation that was mostly CBD with only trace amounts of THC. I contend, as noted elsewhere in this book, that some THC is needed for an individual's endocannabinoid system to reach homeostasis or their wellness balance. This worked for Jessica as it has for others.

"It brought me back to me," she says. "My pain is less. The panic attacks are gone. I'm able to function at home again and be there for my kids and my husband."

Experiencing Epileptic Seizures

Just like some who have a proclivity towards addictions, sometimes we're prone to cognitive issues because of our genetic dispositions. A good friend Tanya had that type of experience. At age 30, this young woman was living a full and active life. Then, she suffered her first seizure.

"It was scary, very scary," Tanya says. "In a public place. I was frightened, embarrassed, and literally did not know what hit me or what to do."

That event led to another and another. She had fainting spells, seizures, and grand mal seizures. It was progressive. It got worse. And doctors did everything they could for her; they tried every medication, every new therapy that came their way. Epilepsy affects nearly 50 million people worldwide. It's not a lottery you want to win. For Tanya, her seizes were triggered by stress, by environmental factors, which meant she usually had seizures in public places. "When I came to, I was usually in an unfamiliar place and I remember the questions they would ask me: What's your name? How old are you? Did you take any medications or drugs?"

Battling the disease, Tanya, like many others, suffered from PTSD from the public seizures, had panic attacks when she heard sirens, and all of it brought her into a deep depression. The medications for the disease were equally bad. They affected her sleep, they dulled her mind, erased parts of her memory, and killed her appetite yet promoted weight gain. Scary drugs, really; they were meant to temper what is considered abnormal brain activity.

As a result, Tanya lost her driver's license for a while. And she spent many hours waiting for or being seen by doctors. She was always looking for answers. Even went to a brain clinic at UCLA to see if they would prescribe medicinal cannabis, which was known to help people suffering from epilepsy, but they turned her down.

Tanya says that on one visit, she met a patient who was suffering from PTSD. He was taking cannabis, and it was controlling his symptoms. "So I used him as a guide and began to create my own wellness plan. I started tracking what my brain was doing using cannabis, and what I saw were only improvements."

Against a doctor's advice, Tanya began to wean herself off of pharmaceuticals. "The first month, my brain was cloudy," she says. And then she gave herself several months to experiment with cannabis doses, to find the right formulation. Soon she started to see improvements. "It helped a lot. And I began to feel better in every way." Tanya became seizure free, having found freedom in medicinal cannabis. What helped her most, she says, is that she was careful with everything she put in her body. "I know my triggers, so I avoid environments or situations which can elevate my anxiety." Mindful of her body, she greatly improved the quality of her life. Now, many years later, Tanya works with me and with others to educate people on the benefits of medicinal cannabis. Together, we are finding people who have similar life-changing experiences and are gathering evidence to further support research for those studying epilepsy and other brain conditions.

Divorce Takes Its Toll

My co-author has a joke he uses in his stand-up act: "Death, taxes, and divorce. Two of these three things suck." I'm divorced so I would say all three are unpleasant. Divorce is something nearly half of the U.S. married population have faced. For those who have gone through it, or are going through it, it's stressful and painful in many ways. Cannabis can help.

Meet John, a typical guy. Average looking, good job, physically active. When I met John, unfortunately, he was struggling because he had been in a long-term relationship that was ending. He was going through a bad divorce, and it was affecting his health and well-being. He tells me, "I was so depressed I couldn't get out of bed. That wasn't me. I never felt that way before."

Like many people in this new age of medicinal cannabis, John heard that cannabis could lift the veil of depression. "Friends were telling me to give it a try," he says. "So I tried cannabis, and it made everything worse."

John's situation is not uncommon. Many people experiment with medicine that can help them, but then the experiments go badly. In fact, John readily admits that he did not know what he was consuming and did not know what he was doing. That's why I tell everyone to get their DNA tested—it's a way to establish a baseline or beginning point. Without a DNA report, we're treating people blindly.

John invested in a 23andMe test, and when the results came in, he showed them to me. Sure enough, he had markers that indicated that he was prone to depression. His divorce had triggered the genes, and he was depressed. Moreover, he was consuming a high-THC, indica-dominant hybrid. John didn't know anything about the product; he just knew it was good cannabis. However, it was something that recreational users would experiment with for its mind-altering properties. That particular indica-dominant cultivar is loaded with the terpene myrcene and exacerbates the feeling of depression, making the condition even worse.

I reviewed John's genetic profile and realized he has multiple genotypes associated with increased risk of major depressive feelings. I suggested he modify his protocol to include a balance of THC and CBD as well as changing the terpene profiled to include limonene and linalool. He did and, in a week, he was out of bed. Within a few weeks, he was feeling better, as many of his depression symptoms abated. The cannabis adjustment for John worked. It wasn't a cure all—he still had to go through the divorce and had to deal with those trials and tribulations—but the right formulation allowed him to get out of the funk.

For depression, the chemical imbalance occurs during a process known as neurotransmission. Neurotransmitters release chemicals in our brains that tell us what to think and what to feel. When people are clinically depressed, there is an issue with the way they accept or release specific neurotransmitters that affect mood and personality. It's basically an imbalance in the brain.

This sounds depressing—but it's no joke. Depression hurts. Seek help if you are struggling with depression. I also suggest that people with depression consider consuming a more balanced CBD to THC product because the consumption of high amounts of THC may worsen your depression symptoms. CBD has been shown in studies to be an inverse agonist of THC. In pharmacology, an inverse agonist is a drug that binds to the same receptor as an agonist but induces a pharmacological response opposite to that of the agonist. An agonist increases the activity of a receptor above its basal level, whereas an inverse agonist decreases the activity below the basal level. CBD has been shown in studies to be an inverse agonist of THC. Regardless of how it works, if it works for you is the key question.

My suggestion to everyone is to ask your doctor and follow her advice. And again, seek help. That's the first step.

And if you're getting a divorce, hang in there. Times will get better.

A Veteran Fights PTSD

Men and women in the armed services in this country have some of the most harrowing stories. Not knowing what they have faced, I could not begin to understand what they have to deal with when they come home from serving overseas. Sometimes a vet will ask me for suggestions or information on cannabis use. I usually have some ideas based on the struggles they tell me about.

A case in point is Jim, a veteran of the war in Iraq. From his years of service overseas he has experienced PTSD as well as pain, especially in his joints. This is not uncommon among returning vets.

His original doctor associated with the VA recommended an SSRI (Prozac) to help address the symptoms of PTSD and an opioid for pain.

Jim quickly became dependent on the opioid. If his doctor would've done a DNA test, he would have seen that Jim has several genotypes associated with an increase of opioid dependence. In fact, his DNA report shows he has a gene that has a 61% predisposition to opioid dependence. Doctors, perhaps, would recommend alternatives to opioids if they knew this.

After Jim was able to kick his opioid dependence, he found another doctor who recommended cannabis as an alternative. More doctors are seeing cannabis as a viable treatment protocol.

Jim decided to try cannabis. He went to a dispensary and purchased pre-rolled cannabis that the budtender recommended. Jim remembered the "giggle weed" he tried back in high school, and the budtender recommended a sativa.

When Jim smoked his joint, he began to experience loss of psycho-motor control, which proceeded to make him anxious. That anxiety quickly escalated to a psychotic reaction, which means a person becomes confused about what is real.

Jim's pride did not allow him to communicate his adverse effect, and he thought maybe it was a one-time event. He decided to do it again and had a similar negative experience.

Jim concluded that he was not able to consume cannabis and doubled up on the Prozac instead (which has many chronicled side effects). A friend told him about Endo·dna, and, unhappy with the increased dosage of Prozac, he decided to try the Endo·dna test.

When he received his results, it showed that he had a genetic predisposition to psychotic effects and loss of psychomotor control. The results suggested consuming a more balanced CBD to THC formulation with linalool and beta-caryophyllene. Jim found his formulation and was able to eventually replace his SSRI with his personalized Endo-Aligned formulation, per his doctor's instructions. And it worked. And he enjoys the benefits of this healing plant without worrying that the effects will be anything but beneficial.

Here's a little more science to explain what Jim experienced. Motor control is important for complex tasks like driving. Although THC can impair motor control, there have been some inconsistencies in studies, which may be due to genetic differences among study subjects. Everybody has different levels of sensitivity to THC and CBD, so getting the right balance between the two is required for those people looking to enjoy cannabis recreationally and for those looking for its true health benefits. I coined and trademarked the phrase "Cannabis is Personal" when I started Endocanna Health. For Jim and so many other people, it really is.

Cannabis-Related Psychosis

One day, not long too ago, I was on the phone with a medical doctor who works in a health clinic in New Jersey. Our conversation was interrupted, and the doc asked me to "hold" the phone. On the other end, I heard a lot of yelling and screaming, and then I heard voices of what sounded like a medical team. When the doctor came back, he told me that a patient who had ingested cannabis was experiencing a psychotic break, and he had to be sedated so he could be treated. It was not a usual occurrence, he told me, but does happen from time to time.

My co-author, Brian, a college professor, also told me a similar story about one of his students. He was a bright young man at a prestigious college back East, who one day ended up in the ER—taken there by campus security. The student had smoked some cannabis with a group of friends and after only a few hits, ended up freaking out. Everyone else had a normal recreational experience. But not this young man. And he was reportedly the least experienced recreational user in the group. It was not his first time using cannabis, but that event was his first ever psychotic episode. Again, this is not a usual occurrence but does happen from time to time. By the way, that kid turned out to be fine and graduated and went on to a good career. He stopped with the THC, of course, although today we could advise him differently.

Experiencing Something Like Psychosis

With the last story in mind, I consulted one young woman, Susan, who took a DNA test to determine why she reacted badly when using THC. When she is with friends and they consume edibles, everyone in her group has a good experience. Except for Susan.

"I'm the only one of my friends who freaks out," she says. It's terrible. I have a really negative reaction. I knew something wasn't right." What Susan was experiencing were panic attacks and hallucinations. And she thought she was going crazy. But that was not the case. Her symptoms occurred only when she ingested cannabis. Her DNA test results showed that she had a metabolic predisposition for anxiety. On top of that, she had the psychosis genotype. This meant she had to avoid edibles and high doses of THC, but lower doses of THC would be OK. "It was a relief to have scientific evidence as to why this happens," she says. "Now I know what I can and cannot do."

If you have this info, and this kind of severe reaction happens to you, you have the power to take care of yourself. First, don't panic. Know that those feelings will go away. And then you have to be mindful—use products that have a higher CBD level and titrate down on the THC. Avoid edibles if you have a slow metabolism. You just need to modify how you consume cannabis.

Susan is a slow metabolizer. She feels the effects much slower, but when it hits, it's intense and lasts longer. Her consumption also triggers that psychosis gene—so she starts hallucinating. People with this condition end up in the hospital. Dosing matters. Formulations matter. For Susan, this means consuming a more balanced formulation, so she avoids negative outcomes and experiences positive effects without fear.

Want to know more? I get that. This is interesting stuff, and luckily, it's not common. Psychosis from cannabis generally causes delusions, which are strong beliefs that are not based in reality and are often inconsistent with the user's actual beliefs. These beliefs can range from finding great meaning in everyday objects to even believing that oneself is God.

Psychotomimetic effects are drug-induced increases in states that resemble psychosis. They can include symptoms such as delusions and hallucinations. Whether you experience psychotomimetic effects is highly dependent on THC dose, as I explained a few paragraphs back. At a high enough dose, virtually everyone will experience some psychotomimetic effects. However, some people have predisposing factors that make them more sensitive to these effects and they will experience them even at typical THC doses. This is likely due to genetic differences that cause increased dopamine signaling in the striatum after THC use.

THC can cause psychotomimetic effects in some people, but it is important to understand that these effects are temporary and will wear off with other THC effects. Many other drugs are capable of causing psychotomimetic effects, including hallucinogens, stimulants, and certain opioids.

Psychosis really is a symptom of multiple illnesses, and there is not one cause. Still, there is a risk that cannabis use will cause psychosis. And different people have different levels of risk of psychosis from cannabis use. A person's risk of experiencing cannabis-related psychosis depends on factors from their genetics and environment.

For example, having the AKT-1 gene, along with other factors, can lead to a psychotic episode. And this only happens, in this case, when you are high.

To sum up the scary stuff, in order to avoid psychosis from cannabis use, consume products that do not have high levels of THC. Use one with a higher amount of CBD. It is also important to consume cannabis products formulated with the appropriate terpenes in order to avoid cannabis-induced psychosis. Really, truly, this is the best reason to have your DNA tested. Your test is an insurance policy. The risk for cannabis-related psychosis is low, but it can be avoided altogether with a little more knowledge of your genetic make-up. Take the test!

Prostate Cancer and Cannabis

When Pete was diagnosed with prostate cancer at age 70, he underwent regular treatments, but after three years, he was doing well. He had read about the benefits of cannabis and went to a dispensary and began using a full extract of cannabis oil. Peter was taking a formulation in a suppository that measured out at 71% THC and 55% CBD oil, and he took it three times a day.

It didn't help. In fact, he was losing weight, and losing sleep, and was getting worse. And he was getting depressed. He stopped doing many outside activities, which did not help either. I was all too happy to help him figure it out, of course, because I was sure he should be getting some benefit. His DNA test showed me that he would do better with a sublingual and with less THC. He also had the genetic marker for a psychotic reaction to THC, which explained his anxiety and inability to sleep. So, with my help, he titrated down. In addition, we included a terpene profile change in the formulation he was using, Not long after, his mood changed. He started to sleep. And he became active again, even feeling up to going out on hikes, a favorite pastime for him. Here again, we knew there would be a cannabis benefit but needed to look at a genetic profile to figure out the right formulation and to decide how best to administer the medicinal product. Most of all, it helped Pete avoid a more serious adverse reaction—something that could have happened if he continued using the initial full-extract product he self-administered.

Peter's story is, in a sense, a warning for others. Most people do not have the gene marker that indicates psychosis is possible with THC ingestion. But a few people do have that marker. The way to find out, of course, is to have your DNA tested.

Is Impulsivity a Side Effect?

Some people do stupid things when they get high. That's not surprising; cannabis relaxes the mind. Anxiety is one of the most common reasons people give for using medical marijuana. It's probably why most of us gravitate towards it when in high school. Stressful times promote a need for stress reduction. In one study, researchers at Washington State University found that some 58 percent of users cited this as their reason for using cannabis. That was second only to pain, for which nearly 61 percent said was the reason for their use. Other scientific evidence shows that the drug can help reduce anxiety. According to a study published in the *Journal of Affective Disorders,* cannabis reduced anxiety by more than 57 percent of users who were tested.

The endocannabinoid system regulates activation of a brain region called the amygdala. The amygdala controls your physiological response to stress and feelings of anxiety. In particular, an endocannabinoid called anandamide can regulate how much your amygdala is activated by stress. Anandamide levels in the amygdala are controlled by a metabolizing enzyme called FAAH. I highlight how this works elsewhere in the book, but remember, a person's own genetics affect these activations.

There's also a genetic marker that some people have that can cause some bad decision making. When stressed, these people might make some bad choices.

This guy that I know, Joe, tells me that cannabis makes him impulsive. For some people, jumping the gun is a regular thing. They have a predisposition to impulsivity.

Joe realized this was a real problem at a holiday office party for a new job he had. He was nervous around his new boss, so before the party, he took a few hits, thinking it would make him less nervous. Then he had a few drinks. Then came the brownies. You get the picture. The cliché is that he would end up wearing a lampshade. It was nothing that silly, but his impulsivity nearly cost him his job.

Such impulsiveness is an adverse effect of THC. Impulsivity is the tendency to act without fully considering the consequences of your choices and actions. You're likely acting impulsively if you make choices quickly that you're prone to question or regret later. But here's the kicker: THC will not increase everybody's impulsivity in the same way. Some people seem more susceptible to this effect than others. Genetic variants in the dopamine system (such as DBH, which is responsible for metabolizing dopamine) may influence your susceptibility to increased impulsivity from THC.

The next day, Joe's work friends called him and laughed about his impulsive behavior. Joe felt an overwhelming sense of regret when he remembered the look on his boss's face while he was telling stories about his college days. That night he also maxed out a credit card, buying online an expensive cruise package. He had promised his fiancée he would cool it when it came to overdoing it—so she did not speak to him for days after.

Joe was able to recover from his behavior at the holiday party, fix the credit card issue, and apologize numerous times until his fiancée forgave him. He also swore off cannabis altogether. Joe assumed he outgrew pot and figured all cannabis would make him act immaturely and impulsively. But the story does not end there.

Later that year, Joe was diagnosed with Crohn's disease. He spent months researching therapies to help with the chronic pain. Many of his friends in online forums and Facebook groups suggested cannabis therapy to help manage his symptoms. Joe wanted to use cannabis again for that reason, but obviously, he was afraid he would make choices he'd regret later. Joe had a friend on Facebook who also managed her Crohn's symptoms after understanding her genetics. She turned to me, to my team, and we helped her use cannabis to live more comfortably. Joe did the same. He was able to discover his genetic predispositions to adverse events with THC—and learned why it triggered his impulsive behavior. He found help and was able to use CBD properly to treat the Crohn's symptoms.

His story, like those of many others I am recounting, shares a similar theme. People who experience adverse effects when using cannabis and keep using it are not listening to their bodies. On the other hand, those who swear off cannabis might be avoiding adverse effects, but they are losing out on medication that could help them live more comfortably. I'm a proponent of cannabis for this reason. Cannabis can safely be used recreationally, but in moderation—in the way that people might enjoy a good bottle of wine. But the medicinal benefits should not be downplayed. For many people, cannabis is a lifesaver.

Cannabis and Neurodegenerative Conditions

Neurodegenerative conditions include Alzheimer's, multiple sclerosis (MS), Parkinson's, Huntington's, and other different neuromuscular atrophies. All are quite horrible. So why are people afflicted with these diseases? According to research, genetic mutations, injury, and age seem to be the main culprits.

Cannabis helps alleviate symptoms of these conditions in two ways:

1. It helps to reduce spasms and other symptoms that are controlled through the CB1 channel, where THC plays a modulating role by stimulating the endogenous retrograde neurotransmitters.

2. THC reduces microglia, which are supposed to protect cells, but prolonged release of microglia actually deteriorates neurotransmitters. However, CBD has shown in studies to reduce the production of microglia.

The clear conclusion is that a person needs the whole plant to work as a neuro-protectant. I started Endocanna Health to check genetic predispositions of cannabis users to determine what is right for each individual, including terpene profiles. There are numerous studies to support this, and an end to marijuana prohibition will foster new research as well as new and better strains of medicinal plants.

Cannabis and Multiple Sclerosis

Some medical conditions can cause a lot of things to go haywire, and life then becomes difficult to manage. For Henry, a single dad who has three kids, cannabis helps him navigate the symptoms of multiple sclerosis.

Henry has three kids. His eldest son, Billy, is a few years older than his twin daughters, Becky and Laura. Henry works at the local elementary school as a teacher's assistant. He runs several parent-teacher activities in the community and volunteers to help set up the Math Marathon Study Festival in the gymnasium every year. He's an involved dad. Something we all should be (those of us who are dads).

As an adult, Henry was diagnosed with multiple sclerosis. At first, his symptoms were manageable, but they soon became more debilitating. He suffered from impaired vision, chronic pain, tremors, and fatigue. Mornings were particularly difficult. Luckily, a neighbor took over driving the kids to school. Other symptoms, like shaking hands, made it hard for this dad to help his kids with their homework.

"I had to go outside to use my cannabis vape pen," he says. It helped sometimes. But not often enough. Henry only used cannabis when he really needed it. He didn't like getting high, but he hadn't been able to find another solution to manage the acute onset of his symptoms.

"I smoked cannabis for relief, but the results were inconsistent," he says. Sometimes he felt good after using the vape, and sometimes he felt awful, the cannabis having little or no effect. That truly was frustrating because when the cannabis use worked, it worked really well for him.

Unfortunately, cannabis affected his memory too. "I would be helping my son with his math homework and would take a break to use the vape. But then I tried to help Billy work on his math and couldn't remember how the problems should be solved. I even had trouble after reading the equation solutions and could not help him complete the problems."

Henry felt like he lost his ability to think critically. He lost his edge, his sharpness. He would stare at a blank page and feel like he was in a fog.

Cannabis was helping relieve his MS symptoms, but not always. And sometimes it blanked his mind, but not always. Frustrated with the inconsistency of the cannabis products he was using, Henry decided to find out why. He did some research and learned that he couldn't count on a specific cannabis strain to deliver the same experience or effectiveness every time.

However, Henry did come across an online forum where a woman with MS shared her experience because of Endo·dna. My company experts were able to find a cannabis product that was genetically aligned to her unique health goals. Henry then sought our help too. He used his 23andMe DNA results to get a personalized wellness plan. He took that information to his doctor, and they agreed on a specific formulation that would be delivered in a sublingual spray.

His new cannabis therapy routine works much better. Henry got rid of the vape and used a spray as needed. He felt better when his symptoms were under control and he was no longer cognitively impaired. His kid's math homework? Problem solving was no longer a problem. Henry did the math.

Butter Fingers and Two Left Feet

People who cannot dance are said to have two left feet. Add cannabis to that condition, and that lack of dexterity becomes epic. Cue
sound cut: "I can't dance, I can't sing" by Phil Collins, right? Now
that does not apply to my friend Andrea, who is not a bad dancer,
but she does experience a movement-related adverse effect of THC.
Andrea smokes a joint and immediately after the THC kicks in, she
has trouble standing up and even speaking. Soon after, she loses
psychomotor control. Psychomotor control is commonly referred to
as coordination. It involves the careful alignment of both thinking
and physical movement. You use psychomotor control in everyday
tasks, like driving, walking, and chewing.

A few years ago, Andrea celebrated ten years as an accountant.
Although she loved her career, she felt a calling to learn more about
environmental sustainability, so she decided to go back to school for
a second bachelor's in environmental science. Andrea took classes
at night on a part-time basis for four years. In 2019, she graduated
with honors. Andrea's coworkers threw her a party to celebrate her
new achievements. They hosted a bonfire on the beach, brought their
favorite snacks, and set up a volleyball net in the sand.

Marcy, Andrea's best friend and co-worker, knew Andrea had
worked hard to get her second degree. Marcy always volunteered to
pick up Andrea's kids from school when Andrea had to meet with an
advisor or run to campus unexpectedly.

Just before sunset, Marcy and Andrea took a walk along the board-walk, and Marcy took out a joint and lit it.

"I bought these from the dispensary downtown," she said. "The budtender said these are his personal favorites." Andrea, who hadn't smoked cannabis since her twenties, took a large inhale and coughed. We all know that experience.

Almost immediately, Andrea stopped walking and sat down on the boardwalk. Marcy asked if she was okay, but Andrea couldn't seem to speak. Instead, she motioned for Marcy to pass the joint. But Andrea couldn't hold onto the joint when Marcy passed it. She dropped it in the sand. When she picked it up, she dropped it again.

Marcy, sensing Andrea was having an adverse reaction, put the joint out and insisted they sit together until Andrea felt better. After a long while, Andrea started to feel like herself again, and she was relieved that she could stand up on her own. They walked back to the bonfire, but Andrea didn't feel much like celebrating anymore.

For the rest of the evening, Andrea wondered why she had such a bad reaction to the joint. She had smoked cannabis before but never had such trouble with her motor skills.

The next morning, Andrea did some research online. She learned loss of motor control can happen for those who use cannabis recreationally or medicinally. Genetics again.

A few weeks later, Andrea and Marcy met at the beach again. Andrea told Marcy about how her genetics played a role in her adverse reaction to the joint they shared at her party. Moreover, she told Marcy she was able to find the right products for her genotype.

After using high-THC cannabis, she had an adverse effect, but then she found a product with a more balanced ratio of THC and CBD that had a different terpene profile. If you are aware of it, then you can counter the effect that high THC can have on coordination and physical balance.

Today Macy does not worry about losing her coordination or mobility as an adverse event from THC. Genetics can help you coordinate cannabis use as well. Not sure that cannabis can help with the dancing. But maybe science will one day figure that out too.

Aggression and Depression

Jacob, a colleague, uses cannabis for pain and inflammation. He came to me one day after an incident where he was smoking some flower and then became overly aggressive while playing a new video game. People might want to blame video games for it, but Jacob experienced aggressive behavior as an adverse effect of THC. Aggressive behavior is behavior directed at yourself, objects, or others, intending physical or mental harm. The event scared him because it was too familiar. He was diagnosed with a mood disorder as an adult. After his diagnosis, Jacob struggled to find medication or therapies that worked for him. He tried a few different strategies with a therapist, but it was not enough, and he continued to look for ways to cope with his irregular and unpredictable moods.

Eventually, Jacob found a daily routine that he liked. He woke up early, did a quick exercise routine while his coffee was brewing, and went to work at the local sanitation department for his regular eight-hour shift. Jacob and his colleagues were a close-knit group, so he enjoyed his shifts most of the time. When he got home, Jacob usually played video games before dinner. It was his favorite way to relax after a long day.

On one drive home, Jacob was feeling irritable. We all have those days. Maybe we're overworked, or tired. My co-writer says it's grouchy sitcom dad syndrome—the kind of frustration exhibited on television shows like *The Flintstones*, or more modern shows like *Seinfeld* and

Curb Your Enthusiasm. Anyway, Jacob stops by a dispensary on his way home and asks the budtender for a product to help improve his mood. You can imagine that that's what a dispensary is for.

He left the dispensary with a cannabis strain he'd never tried before and a bag of gummies. The cannabis kind, not the Halloween sugary good stuff. Jacob smoked the cannabis as soon as he got home and he felt great. He played video games for a few hours and felt less irritable than he did after work. He put on a funny movie and then fell asleep early and easily.

The next day, after work, Jacob hopped online to play a new video game with his co-worker. He ate a few gummies, ordered a pizza, and settled down on the couch.

He lost the first round of the game and started to get annoyed. When he lost the second and third rounds, he cursed into his headset and threw his controller at the wall. It left a dent, which made the guy even more angry. It took Jacob nearly twenty-four hours to feel better.

A few days later, Jacob was considering stopping by the dispensary again, but he didn't want to get angry, which he thought could have been an adverse reaction to THC. He was curious if the gummy had prompted his outburst. So he did some research online.

Jacob found Endo·dna and uploaded his Ancestry.com DNA results. He received his Endo·Decoded Report instantly and was surprised to discover his aggressive feeling and behavior were genetically indicated. Now that was something to be pissed about. However, he received an Endo-Aligned suggested formulation, Jacob found the right product with the right balance of THC and CBD, and that changed his entire experience with cannabis.

The guy even went a step further. He started seeing a therapist again and a psychiatrist and shared his Endo·Decoded Report with them. With that information, and also with Endocanna's Drug to

Drug Interaction Report, Jacob was able to consult about the medicinal benefits of cannabis with his team of healthcare professionals and found help for his situation.

Though experiencing aggression as a side effect of THC is rare, if you share Jacob's genotype, you may experience a similar effect.

This was true for my friend Mark. We would paint together and sell our work and the work of others who worked with us in the same art studio. Mark is a good guy. He liked to smoke a lot. He told me he had some issues with smoking because he smoked too much. Later, when we were in a cannabis business, it did not seem to be a problem. We had our delivery service, and Mark was the head of delivery. But then problems developed. During that time, I started noticing that Mark would get aggressive when he would consume a certain amount, and then he really started acting strange, and it culminated in some bad moments. One time I remember he started cursing and yelling at one of the investors in our business. The next day, he was apologetic and didn't feel the same things that made him angry the day before.

I started looking at this pattern; Mark was experiencing aggressive behavior. I've always thought of cannabis as being a peaceful thing. People usually don't smoke cannabis and want to get in a bar fight. But like Jacob, who I mentioned above, and Mark, there is a very small population of people that have a genotype that is associated with aggressive behavior and also impulsive behavior. A gene called HTR2B together with the dopamine beta hydroxylase (DBH) enzyme is associated with a susceptibility to increased impulsivity after consuming THC. Together with these genes, THC misused can create somewhat of a storm.

I've witnessed this maybe one other time. I was consuming cannabis because it would relax me and let me escape the abuse that I had in my house, and all of that other angst from my early years. My parents, when they would find my stash, would tell me that I was angry and hostile when I was on this shit. The funny thing is that I was angry and hostile because of all mental abuse and everything I was going through. Cannabis was the main reason I could really chill. Sometimes perception means something.

One's environment may be the cause of stress, and may lead to anger issues. But in the case of Jacob, maybe it's those video games, or for Mark, maybe it's work issues. Maybe there is another reason to find out what makes you tick (at the genomics level).

The Sheriffs Get It

As a teen and then as a young man, I was no friend of law enforcement, but now I count the Los Angeles Sheriff's Department's deputies as my latest recruits in the effort to teach people about cannabis-use benefits. This is the same sheriff's department that had a long and checkered history with crime and a long-standing feud with the LAPD, both of which had connections to organized crime. Watch old movies of the mean streets of L.A., and you'll catch a glimpse of a world that was realistically captured in the films *Chinatown* and *L.A. Confidential.*

A few years back, the L.A. Sheriff's Department raided my dispensaries and broke them down. We were put out of business because California had not quite gotten its act together in terms of regulating cannabis distributors, and somebody got the idea to temporarily shut down distributors since cannabis was still a federally controlled substance. My places were literally raided by the cops and the cannabis seized. It was like a scene out of the movies.

Recently, however, my feelings for the department have changed. At their invitation, I met with a group of sheriff deputies and other local law enforcement to discuss cannabis benefits.

There's nothing like meeting up and having a sit-down with the same people you were always ducking away from. In the old days, when kids used to cruise around, listening to music and smoking weed, law enforcement could put a damper on things. Times have changed. Legalization in some states; normalization in others. Decriminalization across the country just on the horizon.

So, I met with the cops. I talked about CBD, THC, how both work to heal pain, inflammation, alleviate depression, help with sleep, and provide a myriad of other benefits. I received a genuinely warm response. After I give a talk, I usually have a dozen people waiting to chat with me personally. The L.A. sheriffs were no different. They were interested for themselves and were looking to see how it would benefit their families and communities. Equally important, they wanted me to come back again, to educate more deputies about this fledgling industry.

Thinking about that talk, and my earlier history, makes that entire experience seem so surreal. These are the guys who raided my dispensaries. They once arrested me and my people for trying to help people. Now I'm talking to them, helping them figure out how to help people. In fact, one officer wanted me to go around to speak at schools to talk about cannabis, why it is medicinally beneficial, and why using it without medical authorization could be dangerous. They wanted me to give talks that provided an honest assessment of what can happen. It's a talk I give to many different groups and people. Cannabis can be used recreationally, but to use it medicinally requires expertise and knowledge.

Since my talk, many of the officers have contacted me. These people have sought individual help. One wanted advice on how he could help his mother who was suffering with cancer. Another contacted me for his sister who was stricken with glaucoma. Another sought help for a kid who had ADHD. My favorite story involves one sheriff's wife who wanted help with their dog. I get that a lot. Pets are people too, right? I made recommendations—they worked—and now they have CBD formulations for themselves and their hound.

Not Sleeping, Not Feeling Well

I have many stories. Too many about cancer because it's way too prevalent and because for years, the only people who could use cannabis were cancer patients. It was socially acceptable for them, as far as the authorities were concerned.

That brings me to Joan, a middle-aged woman who was suffering from cancer and was undergoing chemotherapy. She contacted me because the chemo was making her feel ill in many ways. And so she tried cannabis to see if it would help her—but it made her uncomfortable, anxious, and instead of helping her rest, it made sleeping that much harder.

"I can't take it anymore," she told me. "I have so much anxiety, I'm not sleeping, and I'm not feeling good."

Many are in the same boat as Joan. Cannabis does not seem to do for them as advertised, and in some cases, it seems to make chemo's side effects even worse. I told Joan I was glad she contacted me. I had seen this before and thought I could help.

First, we needed to see Joan's DNA profile. Joan took a DNA test. Her profile showed that there was a high likelihood she would have a negative reaction to cannabis. In other words, cannabis with a high THC content would trigger her anxiety. It is unlucky but not tragic since there is a work-around to this problem.

I helped Joan find a formulation that gave her the benefits that came with CBD oils but also limited THC to an amount that would not trigger anxiety. Then, after the formulation appeared to be help-ing Joan and was not making her anxious, I helped her find a second formula that would help with sleep. So, she had two formulations—one for daytime and one for nighttime. The second formulation had a little more THC—just enough to act as a calming agent; one that helped Joan ease into sleep. "Sleeping helps. It made treatment easier to take and made me feel better," she says.

The result of sleeping well, getting the benefits of cannabis, may have actually helped Joan recover from cancer. A PET scan showed that the tumor had shrunk 65 percent.

Cancer is like a fighter on the ropes. It's waiting for an opening, for a place where it can get in its punches. It hides, ducks for cover, lays under a protein layer, keeping the immune system from detecting it. And then it consumes and replicates, destroying good cells. Studies suggest that THC helps reprogram gene receptors to control cancer replication. In effect, with the right amount of THC, the cancer cell eats itself and does not attack other cells. The body wants to heal itself; Patch Adams and many other practitioners have known this.

In light of what we know about cancer and other debilitating condi-tions, people need to have some THC if they want the true benefits of cannabis. So, they can ingest CBD with trace amounts of THC during the day when they don't want to be sedated. Then, at night, they can up the level of THC to help calm the body and stimulate sleep. You're still consuming trace amounts, but it's at a slightly higher level. And the amount is increased gradually to keep a person who is susceptible to anxiety from experiencing a negative reaction. If this is you, then you need to understand the genetic expression of anxiety. You do not need to stimulate your body; you just need a small amount of THC to produce a calming effect. Thus, sleep, with its special healing power, can be produced by adjusting the terpene profile.

There is a science behind cannabis and sleep quality, and familiarity with these concepts is most beneficial to someone who suffers from poor sleep issues or who wants to find ways to develop more restful sleep patterns.

More About Sleep

Some people really have a problem with sleep. Some people take medication so they can sleep, but even when sedated, you are not getting your REM sleep. People who do not get enough sleep at night sleepwalk around, fatigued, during their waking hours. They're not mentally sharp. Like zombies, right?

My new friend named Jen is a good case in point. "Tell my story," she says when I tell her I'm writing this book. Here it is: Jen shares a vape with her best friend and forgets where she is and what day it is. That's her story. OK, there's more.

Forgetting stuff is an adverse effect of THC. Working memory requires the brain to temporarily store and use information. It's important for daily reasoning and decision-making tasks, like reading, holding a conversation, and doing simple math problems in your head. Being tired doesn't help either.

Jen set up a Skype session with a new healthcare provider. She told the doctor about her experience with the vape pen. She relayed her anxiety about smoking to relax at night—because cannabis use helped her sleep but not always. The doctor told her that genetics could be used to achieve the optimal therapeutic experience with cannabis. She got tested, got results with recommended suggestions, and the results were excellent. She found a formulation that worked. Gone was the memory impairment from too much THC, and she felt more relaxed at night because the results were consistent and reliable.

With a doctor's help, she found she could use cannabis products safely with the prescription medications she needs for sleep.

So why did cannabis affect her sleep? For some people, introducing high-THC products into their metabolic systems is like consuming too much alcohol. You may get groggy or sleepy, and might actually fall asleep, but the brain is still active. You don't sleep well because the activity being triggered in your brain is not letting you get restful sleep. This happens to a lot of people with childhood trauma or PTSD. When that PTSD is triggered—which can happen with large amounts of THC—it will likely increase anxiety, making it very hard to relax and rest. A lot is happening there. People who are stressed or anxious have trouble sleeping, and sometimes they try to self-medicate by using or ingesting a large amount of weed. A large consumption of THC can make you pass out. But it is unlikely the result will be a good night's sleep.

I know that this can be mitigated if an affected person uses a formulation with less THC and a terpene profile that includes myrcene, linalool, and trepiline. Find cannabis that has more of an indica-dominant profile versus a sativa-dominant profile, and better sleep is likely. That's not a prescription, but it is a formula that works for most.

For Jen, and people like her, finding the right amount of THC with the correct terpene profile leads to a good night and good sleep. And sweet dreams. OK, I cannot promise sweet dreams, but in my experience, the right formulation helps with sleep.

The Rocker Catches Some Zs Too

Sleep is so important, so I have one more story to share about it. Working towards ending cannabis prohibition and helping people find new uses for this ancient medicine has given me the opportunity to meet many people. In fact, I was lucky to become friendly with a famous rock and roll artist from the 1970s and 1980s. Meeting him was fortuitous for both of us. He suffered from Parkinson's but luckily was able to go through stem cell replacement therapy in Europe, which has helped ease his symptoms. Unfortunately, he fell and broke a neck vertebra and later became addicted to the opioid medications he used to fight the pain.

I did a swab test on my new friend and with his DNA report was able to help him find some formulations that would not trigger his dependence genes. I made him a nighttime and daytime formulation, and with those he was able to stop using opioids and other drugs. It worked so well, beyond even what I had hoped for. "I am sleeping, man," he told me on a recent visit to his Hollywood home. That was big news because he was suffering from a sleep disorder and, for nearly 30 years, rarely found rest. Many people who suffer from sleep issues, like the rocker and the others I have written about, can be helped with CBD and THC.

Few things are better at healing what ails the body than a good night's rest. Unfortunately, that's easier said than done when a person suffers from a condition that causes anxiety. Many diseases, aside from pain and their usual symptoms, also cause stress and anxiety. Stressful treatments can lead to depression, which also causes stress. A lot of stress. Altogether, this prevents sufferers from experiencing high quality sleep.

High quality sleep involves exactly what it sounds like: getting a good night's sleep! There are many factors of high quality sleep, such as the amount of time you sleep, the number of times you wake up during the night, and the amount of time it takes to fall asleep. Maintaining high quality sleep is extremely important to remaining productive and keeping a healthy body.

My relationship with this new friend remains an ongoing thing. My team developed formulations specifically for him—working with his physicians to make sure there would be no interactions. He reduced his intake of prescription medication and told me he was able to sleep through the night. He started working again and recording music. One day, at his house, he shared some unreleased music he was working on with me. I felt like part of his crew.

This rocker, when he was unwell or in need of achieving homeo-stasis, was going through a very dark period. It's a time when many creative people like him cannot work and do not produce art. That changed after we found the right formulation. "Your juice helped me connect with my life again," he told me. "My sense of purpose came back, and I can write again." At that point, he asked me if I wanted to hear his new music. It is one of the perks of my business and life—helping someone find their voice and creativity.

There I am in this rock legend's living room. There's a couch and an ottoman. He's lying there, with a window to his garden at his back. He's in full rocker mode, in persona, dressed in his iconic clothes. I'm sitting next to him, shoulder to shoulder. He has this look in his eye, one that gleams, and he asks me: "Want to hear my new song?"

That moment is surreal. The song is raw. Not recorded in the studio, but his voice sounds amazing. And on the couch, he is singing along. Not full out, but he is singing. It's amazing..

He then shakes my hand with both of his. "Thank you so much for helping me," he says.

I was grateful for something that was priceless. I never could imagine I would have this. I was a poor immigrant, a stoner, and small-time dealer, and here I was, helping one of my all-time favorite musicians find his music. All of that was a result of the therapeutic properties of cannabis and my long history promoting it.

I wish I could tell you more about my work with this legend. It's a high point for me. Where all the roads I have been on in this life come together. More than satisfying. It was vindicating, justifying, and legitimizing.

It was a moment where I could reflect on how far I have come. Then I called my dad. I wanted him to be proud...and wanted to remind him that he kicked me out of the house for using weed.

Programmed for Wellness

It's all about genes. Genetics are your foundation. Everything else is built on that. Since the secrets of genomes have been unlocked, science has taken a step forward. As a result, the future is very bright.

In the meantime, it's time to use what we already know. We need to utilize information from our genes and the genes of the plants we consume medicinally. The point is that each person can find homeostasis—the balance—that equates to well-being. What works for one might not work for another. But what works can be discovered. The goal is to get you back to being yourself, and your genetics is your road map to get you there.

Today you can know your endocannabinoid system profile, and knowing it can help you avoid adverse reactions when using CBD and THC formulations and products. In earlier days, for thousands of years, in fact, using natural medicines was guesswork. But now we know where to put in the work; where to look for information that will help each of us find what will work for us.

Today genetic predispositions do not lock you into a rigid or set course of treatment. Genetics indicate a propensity only—maybe it's only half of the equation. Maybe it is something like your height, for example—you can't change that—but how you use that knowledge informs your epigenetic path. The path is the expression of your genetic predisposition—DNA acts as a blueprint showing your predispositions. The consumables you put into your body can actually trigger an epigenetic response. The response is the expression of your blueprint or the expression of your predisposition. The expression of those genes can be known and can lead to many wellness benefits.

Using that information, and using information from your environment, from your lifestyle, allows you the chance to enhance your overall situation or to avoid unnecessary complications. Moreover, based on this collective information, on the feedback data we receive from our partners and our patients, we will be able to observe how all of these factors play a role in wellness. So, over time, as we learn even more, medical practitioners can advise their patients on the formulations that are best based on each individual's disposition.

Today, so many people are reporting back to us on what they are finding, and this is helping us understand how genetics play a role in wellness. In turn, we can provide more people with information that relates specifically to their unique genotypes. One cannot change their genes, but we can identify how their genes express themselves in certain environments, and that will lead to untold benefits.

The future also looks bright because of education. In other words, as people learn more about the benefits of cannabis, the stigma once associated with its use is abating. No longer are people looked down upon, or frowned upon, for using a natural and unprocessed medicinal herb.

The Right Path

People's perspectives change when they acquire new knowledge. This is my mission: to educate people about cannabis and to help them use that knowledge. Cannabis for me was never about getting high. I always understood that there was more to it. I knew this intuitively. I knew this through my own experience. And the more I learned about it, the more I wrote about it, and the more I spoke about it, the more I became convinced that I was on the right path.

If you are on this path too, then know that we have a lot more to learn about the benefits of cannabis and the endocannabinoid system and how natural medicines can help us achieve homeostasis. The knowledge we have is only the beginning of what we will come to know. Currently, there are few human trials relating to cannabis use, and there are not enough studies yet underway, but more are coming. Our knowledge will grow. Until then, our knowledge is but the tip of an iceberg, and what we will learn is the rest of that iceberg, the submerged part covered by the sea. There are over 140 different cannabinoids and 80 different terpenoids, and how they come together, how they collaborate, and how they ultimately interact has yet to be discovered and explored.

Until then, you can join me and thousands of others who are working to figure out how cannabis can benefit our lives. Some people are looking for cures for illnesses or to relieve side effects from more traditional treatments. Others want to enjoy cannabis recreationally but want to do so safely and mindfully.

When I was in the dispensary business, I learned early on that while one product worked for an individual to help relieve pain or inflammation, or help calm them to provide a night's rest, that the same product may not be as effective for someone else or might not work at all. I learned that cannabis is personal. We know that CBD works on pain receptors and acts as an anti-inflammatory. We know that THC is working as an analgesic, and together they are working synergistically, a true balancing act. With that information, we can then personalize the formulations that an individual receives based on their unique genetic profile. We can guide people to better health and a greater feeling of well-being. That's where we are now.

As for medicine in general, the future holds interesting promise because it focuses on individual overall health and wellness. The use of CRISPR, the use of genetic alignment and genetic modification, will augment the ability to individualize. Different types of medications and therapeutics could be made specifically for the individual (almost like 3D printing today). Imagine taking a capsule that includes all of your vitamins, nutrients, cannabinoids and other essential supplements, everything you want, taken in one single capsule a day. A completely individualized healthcare regimen. The idea of having personalized virtual therapeutic treatment is not far off, and that's what Endocanna Health is working on right now.

Healthcare technology will use artificial intelligence to learn about you, so treatment is going to improve over time. Through telemedicine technology, you'll be able to speak to a healthcare professional more conveniently, and they'll be able to use your static and dynamic biomarkers to make personalized recommendation. Even in the moment right now, personalized therapies can be provided to you in real time. And more and more, we're going to see targeted therapeutics using individual cannabinoids on a pharmaceutical level.

We're going to see nutraceutical supplements and parallel path medications. All of these therapies and approaches are going to be used for the betterment of overall health and wellness for specific individuals. Individualized medicine is going to prolong good health, increase longevity, and allow you to live a better life.

ADDENDA

"Always remember that you are absolutely unique.
Just like everyone else."
— Margaret Mead

Len's Theory

These are my bullet-point notes—the outline I developed to better understand and explain what's going on in the body, especially as it pertains to the endocannabinoid system. It's a theory, and I offer it hoping scientists out there can modify or tune it up.

The EndoDNA Stress Response Theory:

- Every human has an endocannabinoid system (ECS), which is a primary regulatory system (much like the nervous system).

- We all have baseline levels of endogenous endocannabinoids; this includes, in the brain, anandamide (AEA), which modulates brain functions like memory, motivation, cognition, movement control, desire, pleasure reward, appetite, and feelings of pain. In the body, 2-AG, another endocannabinoid, affects the immune and digestive systems and helps regulate metabolism, energy, and inflammation.

- The core of the ECS consists of two receptors – CB1 and CB2. CB1 actually is associated with brain function and the central nervous system. CB2 is associated with the digestive system and immune system.

- Ligands are molecules that bind to receptors in the following ways:

- ○ Anandamide (AEA) is an agonist of CB1 (THC mimics the way anandamide works).

- ○ 2-AG is an agonist of CB2 (CBD works in a similar way as 2-AG).

- ○ FAHH regulates the levels of anandamide (AEA). More FAAH produces less anandamide, producing less bliss hormone and a greater propensity to stressors triggering fight or flight responses. (The word "anandamide" originates from the sanskrit "ananda," which roughly translates to "bliss" or "joy," and this is an indication of the cannabinoid's properties as a mood enhancer. Also called N-arachidonoylethanolamine [AEA], anandamide interacts with the body's CB receptors similarly to cannabinoids like THC. It's a neurotransmitter and cannabinoid-receptor binding agent that functions as a signal messenger for CB receptors located in the body. More cortisol is, thus, released, which may increase the body's PH level over time, causing an overactive immune response. This will result in inflammation and the feeling of pain and discomfort. This may also affect gut health over time.

- FAAH rs324420 CC is a risk genotype.

- Anxiety can cluster around worry about a variety of topics, events, or activities, and this worry may shift from one topic to another. One might feel edgy, restless, more likely to tire and fatigue, and have difficulty concentrating. This could include trouble falling asleep or staying asleep and restlessness at night.

- There is marked diversity in how people respond when put in a threatening situation, which activates a part of the brain called the amygdala. The ECS is one of the brain systems that regulates this behavior through a molecule called anandamide. Anandamide is an endocannabinoid whose levels are regulated by the enzyme FAAH. In one study, healthy volunteers who carried the rs324420 "A" allele (low FAAH activity, high anandamide levels) had much less amygdala activation when placed in a threatening situation. They also had a weaker correlation between amygdala activation and trait anxiety, which is a general tendency to perceive situations to be threatening and to respond to such situations with subjective feelings of apprehension and tension.

- More MAGL and DAGL indicates less 2-AG, which can regulate the immune response of inflammation. This is related to prolonged anxiety as well as depressive states (mood disorders).

- Less 2-AG available to regulate the immune response of inflation, and higher a PH due to prolonged cortisol, can lead to chronic autoimmune conditions and other disease states.

The Solution:
- Genetically, we can tell the genotype that has a more prevalent production of FAAH (homozygous) and MAGL, DAGL; and in treatment we can subsidize the endogenous endocannabinoids with phytocannabinoids from cannabis to help restore homeostasis along both of the CB1 and CB2 pathways.

- Two more components of ECS not to ignore are the TRPV1 receptors. THC has shown to be an agonist of these receptors and has a relationship to pain, heat, and blood flow.

About Endocanna Health – My Mission

I am a patient, first of all. I have consumed cannabis as medicine and have a really long and interesting relationship with cannabis for many years since I was a teenager.

Diagnosed with ADD as a child, I was put on a variety of prescription medications that did little to help with my symptoms. Through my own self-discovery, I found cannabis as a helpful alternative to address ADD. Then came years of developing my business career, and my understanding of cannabis, and eventually, it all came together in Endocanna Health. I was dedicated to understanding the role of human gene expression and the endocannabinoid system and co-founded Endocanna Health and set to work creating a DNA test that could identify cannabis strains most likely to help individuals. The result is a breakthrough DNA test powered by a patent-pending super-chip that analyzes unique genomic markers. The information from the DNA test is then turned into a report that gives consumers personalized information about their unique genetic expressions. From there it provides suggestions about cannabis formulations that match what's called individual Endo Compatibility.

Endo Compatibility is an intersection between your unique genetic code and the properties of cannabis plants. Each cultivar has a distinct ratio of CBD to THC along with a host of other cannabinoids and terpenes, each interacting with your body in a unique way. The personalized results from the Endo·dna test are like nothing else on the market, offering consumers an incredible array of science-backed reports about their health and wellness.

When I am asked about what gets me excited to get up each morning, I tell everyone I am super grateful that I get to be a part of the cannabis business in the way that I am. I am just super, super proud and I pinch myself every single day going to work. I'm not really going to work. I'm just doing what I always did. We work, we work hard, but it's amazing. It's an amazing opportunity. With where we're at in history, there is no other industry that had the trajectory in the last few years than that of the cannabis industry. We've gone from complete prohibition to cannabis being legal in more than three-quarters of the country.

Getting personalized cannabis information into the hands of consumers is my mission. Our intent is number one: to avoid an adverse event with cannabis. You can have an optimal experience because *cannabis is personal*. Everybody has a personal experience with cannabis, and two people can take the same exact thing and experience a completely different effect.

So that's really what I want to get out. Everybody needs to understand that cannabis is personal and everybody can have their own personal experience with cannabis and it can be a really good one.

My vision for the future of Endocanna Health promises more breakthroughs in understanding Endo Compatibility. Customers can continue to expect groundbreaking new research and information about their unique DNA that helps them chart their own path to wellness.

Endocanna Health is a biotechnology company committed to helping consumers find the right cannabinoid products to enhance their health and wellness. Using our breakthrough DNA test, Endo·dna, we empower our customers with the ability to take control of their health with access to over 55 different health reports that include suggestions for the best CBD and cannabis products that match their unique genetic code. Cannabis is personal.

Len May Press Appearances

In my role as cannabis advocate and industry insider, I make many public appearances and meet with reporters from all types of media to discuss the benefits of cannabis and the future of the cannabis universe. Below is a cultivated and curated list—information that might be useful for anyone considering seeking work or investing in the industry.

Authority Magazine
Len May of Endocanna Health: "5 Things I Wish Someone Told Me Before I Started Leading a Cannabis Business"

MG Retailer
Cannabliss Retreats Plants Its 420 Seed in a Malibu Mountains Fruit Farm

LA Weekly
The Search for Spirituality and Wellness Is Driving New Image for Cannabis

Rolling Stone
The Rolling Stone Guide to Legal Pot: California

Rolling Stone
Pot-Pairing DNA Tests: Can Genetic Tests Match You With the Best Bud?

Well + Good

Terpenes Are the Unsung Aromatic Heroes of the Cannabis Plant—Here's What You Need to Know

Bloomberg

Weed-Meets-DNA Startup CEO Says Hysterical Market Needs to Relax

Dope Magazine

Cannabis Is Personal: On the Road To Individualized Medicine

Weedmaps

DNA May Show How Marijuana's Effects on Consumers are All in the Genes

Brit + Co

Everything You Need to Know About CBD, the Latest "It" Wellness Ingredient

Can Can Buzz – Canada

Don't Know What Strain? Let Your DNA Be Your Guide

Green Entrepreneur

Green Entrepreneur Top 100 Cannabis Companies

Sacred Plant

The Sacred Plant

Mindful Warrior

Len May: Cannabis and Your DNA on iHeartRadio

The Cannabis Reporter

DNA Sequencing Over-Achieves FDA's CBD Regs

Greener Grass

Len May – Genetics, Cannabis, and You (ep41)

Hemp Connoisseur

Podcasts on EndoCanna Health

Dope Magazine

Cannabis Is Personal: On the Road To Individualized Medicine

Forbes

5 Critical Questions Cannabis Researchers And Producers Are Asking In 2019

Benzinga

Beyond Indica And Sativa: Leafly Launches Graphic Platform For Identifying Cannabis Strains

Cheddar TV

Endocanna Health Bringing Bio-tech to Cannabis Industry (video)

Labroots Cannabis Virtual Conference

Cannabis is Personal! Learn How Your Genetics Play a Big Roll (webinar)

Entrepreneur Magazine/Green Entrepreneur

One Company's Quest to be the 23andMe of Cannabis (podcast)

High on The Hog

E13:Well Worn Genes with Len May CEO EndoCannaHealth (podcast)

Heads Up Health

Episode 32 – EndoCanna Health – Personalizing Medicinal Cannabis with DNA testing (podcast)

Raising Cannabis Capital

0216: EndoCanna Health | Len May (podcast)

Simply Walk The Talk /Josh Holland

Episode 137 – Len May (EndoCanna Health) on Personalised Cannabis + CBD (podcast)

A Playlist: Some Music to Experience

I am often asked from people who know me for my recommendations for albums and suggestions for new things to listen to when kicking back. Cannabis and music likely have been intertwined for thousands of years. I could make a list of several hundred albums, but here's a sampling. Not in any particular order. I purposely have listed only one album per band but obviously could put nearly every Beatles and Led Zeppelin album on the list. Is this the list I would be happy with were I stranded on a desert island? Possibly. But I really don't want to find out.

Jamiroquai – *High Times*
Radiohead – *The Bends*
Zero7 – *Simple Things*
Led Zeppelin – *II*
Beatles – *Abbey Road* (or maybe *Sgt. Pepper's Lonely Hearts Club Band*...)
Muddy Waters – *The Anthology*
Thievery Corporation – *The Richest Man in Babylon*
Pink Floyd – *Dark Side of the Moon*
Beastie Boys – *Check Your Head*
Alice In Chains – *Unplugged*
Black Sabbath – *Paranoid*
Bob Marley – *Exodus*

A PLAYLIST: SOME MUSIC TO EXPERIENCE

Rage Against the Machine – Self-titled

Sade – *The Ultimate Collection*

Rolling Stones – *Made in the Shade*

Guns n Roses – *Appetite for Destruction*

Black Crowes – *The Southern Harmony and Musical Companion*

Cypress Hill – Self-titled

Lauryn Hill – *The Miseducation of Lauren Hill*

Notorious BIG – *Ready to Die*

Prince – *Purple Rain*

Tribe Called Quest – *Low End Theory*

Metallica – *Ride the Lightning*

NWA – *Straight Outta Compton*

Marvin Gaye – *What's Going On*

Stevie Wonder – *Songs in the Key of Life*

John Coltrane – *A Love Supreme*

Eric B. & Rakim – *Paid in Full*

Miles Davis – *Kind of Blue*

Jimi Hendrix Experience – *Are You Experienced*

Wu Tang – *Enter the Wu Tang (36 Chambers)*

Amy Winehouse – *Back to Black*

Red Hot Chili Peppers – *Blood Sugar Sex Magic*

Black Keys – *Brothers*

Chris Cornell – *Songbook*

Robert Johnson – *The Complete Recordings*

Public Enemy – *It Takes a Nation of Millions to Hold Us Back*

Fugees – *The Score*

Mad Season – *Above*

James Brown – *Live at the Apollo*

The Prodigy – *The Fat of the Land*

Jay Z – *The Black Album*

AC/DC – *Back in Black*
Nas – *Illmatic*
Nirvana – *Unplugged*

Some Things to Read

People also say to me, "Len, you're so calm. What's your secret?" After a long pause, letting the asker reconsider the gravity or levity of that question, I tell them that my journey from the underground to corporate boardroom was supported by some *light* reading. More seriously, these are the books that really got me thinking:

The Art of War by Sun Tzu
The Alchemist by Paulo Coelho
The Count of Monte Cristo by Alexandre Dumas
Awaken the Giant Within by Anthony Robbins
The Art of Happiness by Dalai Lama
Think and Grow Rich by Napoleon Hill
The Power of Positive Thinking by Dr. Norman Vincent Peale
How to Win Friends and Influence People by Dale Carnegie
7 Habits of Highly Effective People by Steven Covey
Can't Hurt Me by David Goggins
The Prince by Niccolò Machiavelli
Man's Search for Meaning by Viktor Frankl
The Godfather by Mario Puzo
The Bhagavad Gita by Krishna-Dwaipayana Vyasa
The Power of Now: A Guide to Spiritual Enlightenment by Eckhart Tolle
Outliers by Malcolm Gladwell

The 48 Laws of Power by Robert Greene

Mastery by Robert Greene

The Essential Rumi by Rumi

The Emperor Wears No Clothes by Jack Herer

Genome: The Autobiography of a Species In 23 Chapters by Matt Ridley

The Gene: An Intimate History by Siddhartha Mukherjee

Hacking Darwin: Genetic Engineering and the Future of Humanity by Jamie Metzl

Cannabis and Cannabinoids: Pharmacology, Toxicology, and Therapeutic Potential by Ethan Russo

Cannabis Revealed: How the World's Most Misunderstood Plant is Healing Everything by Bonni Goldstein M.D.

About the Authors

Len May, MCS

As the CEO and co-founder of En-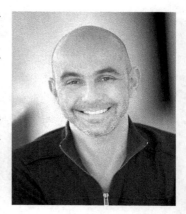
docanna Health, May has more than
25 years of cannabis endocannabinoid system (ECS) and genomics
experience. A pioneer in the medical
cannabis industry, May has been instrumental in shaping the current leg-
islation and culture. He has held past
positions as President of the Cannabis
Action Network and Board Member
and Lifetime Member of California Cannabis Association. May is
the current chair of the CBDIA science board and is a stakeholder
in some of the industry's most iconic brands. His areas of expertise
include the workings of the endocannabinoid system and how genetic
expression plays a role in human experiences. As a certified medical
cannabis specialist, May has an in-depth knowledge of genomics,-
cannabinoids, and terpenes and their interactions with the endocannabinoid system. He holds a Masters of Medical Cannabis and a
certificate in Endocannabinoid Formulation from the Institute for
the Advancement of Integrative Medicine. May is an accomplished
public speaker, having presented on these topics on some of the
world's most prestigious stages in his mission to help educate people
about the healing powers of cannabis. He is the host of the popular
Everything is Personal podcast.

O. Brian Kaufman, PhD

A specialist in corporate and non-profit communications, O. Brian Kaufman is a Professor of English at Quinebaug Valley Community College in Connecticut. At the college he teaches writing and literature and recently developed the state's first Cannabis Studies program. A former editor of *Competitive Utility* and *Project Finance Monthly*, he covered the electric power industry during its deregulation in the late 1990s. With degrees in journalism 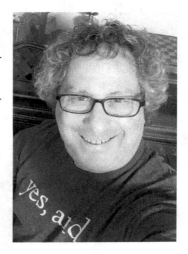 and creative writing and a doctorate in English composition and rhetoric, the former LA-based news reporter, editor, and radio producer covered politics, sports, and business for *The Burbank Leader*, KABC Talkradio, KMNY Money Radio, and others. His latest studies include improvisation and sketch comedy writing with The Second City in Chicago and with the Providence Improv Guild. He continues work on his stand-up career at Flappers Comedy Club in Burbank, CA, and at locations throughout New England.

SUBSCRIBE TO THE

EVERYTHING IS PERSONAL PODCAST

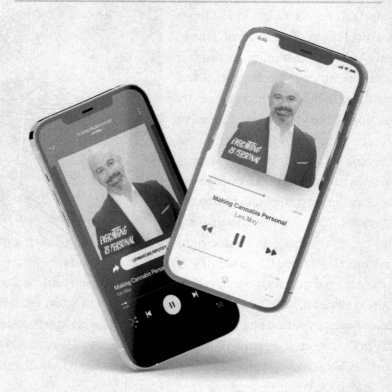

LISTEN ON

SPOTIFY

ITUNES

YOUR
FAVORITE
PLATFORM

CANNABIS, MUSIC, BUSINESS, SOME SCIENCEY STUFF (AND A
TOUCH OF ADD) ALL COME TOGETHER IN ONE AMAZING RIDE

CPSIA information can be obtained
at www.ICGtesting.com
Printed in the USA
JSHW051359280721
17343JS00006B/6